juice+nourish

100 Refreshing Juices and Smoothies to Promote
HEALTH, ENERGY, and BEAUTY

Rosemary Ferguson

THE EXPERIMENT

NEW YORK

JUICE + NOURISH: *100 Refreshing Juices and Smoothies to Promote Health, Energy, and Beauty*

First published in the United Kingdom in 2015 as JUICE by Ebury Press, an imprint of Ebury Publishing.

The Experiment, LLC
220 East 23rd Street, Suite 301
New York, NY 10010-4674
www.theexperimentpublishing.com

This book contains the opinions and ideas of its author. It is intended to provide helpful and informative material on the subjects addressed in the book. It is sold with the understanding that the author and publisher are not engaged in rendering medical, health, or any other kind of personal professional services in the book. The author and publisher specifically disclaim all responsibility for any liability, loss, or risk—personal or otherwise—that is incurred as a consequence, directly or indirectly, of the use and application of any of the contents of this book.

The Experiment's books are available at special discounts when purchased in bulk for premiums and sales promotions as well as for fund-raising or educational use. For details, contact us at info@theexperimentpublishing.com.

Library of Congress Cataloging-in-Publication Data

Ferguson, Rosemary.
  Juice + nourish : 100 refreshing juices and smoothies to promote health, energy, and beauty / Rosemary Ferguson.
    pages cm
  Includes index.
  ISBN 978-1-61519-288-5 (hardcover) -- ISBN 978-1-61519-289-2 (ebook) 1. Detoxification (Health)--Recipes. 2. Self-care, Health--Popular works. I. Title.

  RA784.5.F47 2015
  641.6'2--dc23

                        2015004776

ISBN 978-1-61519-288-5
Ebook ISBN 978-1-61519-289-2

Cover design by Susi Oberhelman
Photography by Nassima Rothacker
Interior design by Two Associates
Food styling by Frankie Unsworth
Styling by Cynthia Inions

Manufactured in China
Distributed by Workman Publishing Company, Inc.
Distributed simultaneously in Canada by Thomas Allen & Son Ltd.

First printing November 2015
10 9 8 7 6 5 4 3 2 1

CONTENTS

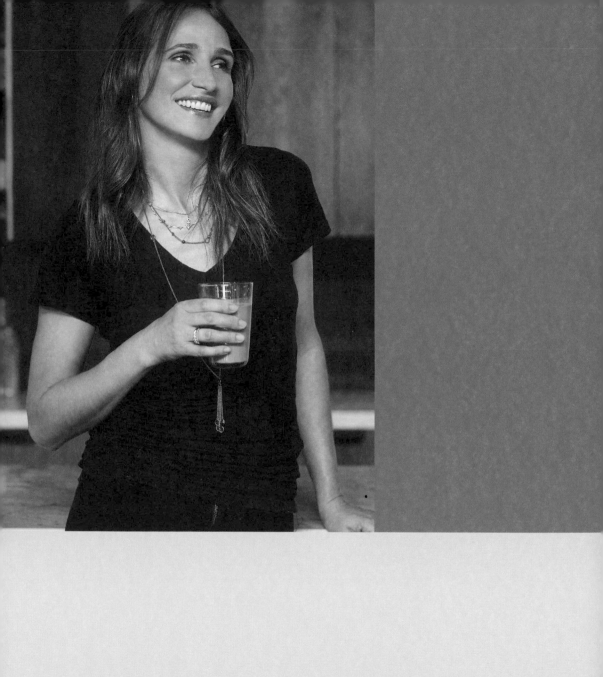

INTRODUCTION

I want this book to inspire you and to help you understand why good nutrition is so important. I am truly passionate about healthy eating, but definitely not evangelical. Small changes can make big differences to your feeling of well-being and energy levels.

I grew up surrounded by complementary medicine, in a family of homeopaths and kinesiologists. My grandmother owned one of the first health food stores in England, inspiring a general awareness of alternative therapies in my family.

I worked as a model for a long time after leaving school, and met some pretty amazing friends and people. While the fashion industry is often blamed for portraying a not-always-positive body image, it is actually where I began to learn about health foods. Most of the people I came into contact with were health conscious and cared about what they ate, and I soon learned about all sorts of wonderful foods and supplements.

Becoming a mom places a very different perspective on food, especially when you're trying to create a balanced meal to satisfy a harsh six-month-old food critic. This often resulted in hilarious trials and errors—or being berated by friends for trying to feed the kids lentils and quinoa, which, for all their early protests, they now love! My long-suffering family became guinea pigs for my food interests way before I decided to pursue it as a career.

I am now a practicing nutritional therapist and naturopath. I write columns for magazines and websites and have a clinic on London's Harley Street. I love my job! Changing the way a person eats can have a profound effect on their health, and I am truly grateful to be able to be a part of that process.

My philosophy is pretty straightforward—I really do believe that a bit of everything is good for the soul, and I'm definitely no angel. I love a good night out, and a bit of junk food now and then.

WHY JUICE & BLEND?

Juices and smoothies are a fantastic way of boosting the intake of nutrients into your diet. I like to think of them as nutrient vehicles.

Raw fruit and vegetables, nuts and seeds are a big part of my diet. The thinking behind eating raw is that when food is cooked, some of the nutrient values are diminished. By juicing or making a smoothie with raw ingredients, the enzymes and other phytochemicals stay intact, and the micronutrients—such as vitamins, minerals, enzymes, and phytonutrients—are preserved in a higher concentration, giving you a more nutrient-dense food. The amount of fruit and vegetables you can pack into a juice means you could get your "5-a-day" in a single glass!

Many of today's chronic conditions such as inflammation, irritable bowel syndrome (IBS), bad skin, and lethargy can be signs of a digestive system that is in trouble. The gut is our tank, where we put the fuel to run our body. It is where absorption of the nutrients that make us work happens, and if it is under par, then we feel under par. Juices can include specific nutrients that are aimed at healing the gut and making it work more efficiently, nutrients such as glutamine, which is fantastic for inflamed stomachs and wonderfully soothing, and is found in cabbage. Not only do juices help resolve problems on the inside, but you will see the benefits on the outside too— glowing skin and bright eyes—while feeling more energetic and vital.

Juice fasting gives the digestive tract a rest and a chance to cleanse the bowel. To help you do this, I have included detox plans for 1, 2, and 3 days. Chewing, eating, and digesting food uses a huge amount of energy every day, so by taking a break and drinking nutrient-rich juices and smoothies for a day or three, you can free up energy for your body to heal other issues.

Both juices and smoothies are alkalizing to the body. The Western diet and stressful lifestyles are very acid forming, creating a condition called acidosis in the body. This is when the pH becomes overly acid and it can wreak havoc in the body, causing premature aging, eczema, mood swings, psoriasis, and fatigue—the list goes on. The body works really hard keeping an alkaline state, so giving it a helping hand by regular juicing and increasing cleaner foods is important. Reducing dairy, red meats, processed foods, alcohol, and coffee and eating a more vegetarian, vegan diet, high in fruits, vegetables, and whole foods, encourages a better acid/alkaline balance.

JUICES VERSUS SMOOTHIES

Juices and smoothies are similar in that they both use raw produce as the base of a nutrient-dense drink. The difference is that juices have the pulp removed and smoothies don't.

Juices are a great vehicle that I use to deliver a boost of phytonutrients, which are extremely easily absorbed by the body.

Smoothies are more substantial than juices and have a higher fiber content because they use the whole fruit or vegetable. Using a blender to make a smoothie also allows you to add in serious nutrient boosters such as seeds, avocados, flaxseed oil, and all sorts of supplemental powders. Simply put all the ingredients into the blender and blend away—it's so easy!

Breakfast is a really important meal, but people often struggle to find time to sit down and eat properly. A smoothie can be a great choice. Substantial and full of nutrition, it is a great start to the day. It is also really useful during detox days if you are struggling with just juices. Smoothies are a way to remain on liquids, but have a little more sustenance to get you through the day.

There have been concerns about the high sugar content in juices and smoothies. This worry mostly comes from shop-bought drinks that are meant to be amazing, but have actually been found to contain a high concentration of sweet fruits, or added sugar, or are made from concentrate or syrups. This can cause all sorts of problems including weight gain, insulin intolerance, and, in serious cases, tooth decay.

It is true that some fruits (and vegetables) have a high natural sugar content, so in the book you will see that I use lots of low-sugar ingredients, such as kale, celery, and cucumber, to counter this. As your taste buds get used to the flavors, you will be able to enjoy juices containing less sugar, opting for the more savory recipes in this book and adding fewer sweet fruits to your own juice and smoothie concoctions.

I also use many fruits that have a high soluble fiber content. Soluble fiber does not get removed during the juicing process, and it slows the absorption of any sugars into the bloodstream and therefore avoids a sugar spike. You can always have a handful of seeds with your juice as this slows absorption too.

A lot of the juices in this book are actually aimed at balancing your blood sugar and helping any insulin intolerance issues. A stable energy level is the ideal, and that is what this book is hoping to achieve.

Another problem with some store-bought smoothies and juices are that they are also pasteurized, meaning they have been heated to get rid of bacteria. Unfortunately this also means that a lot of the goodness has been removed too. There are lots of juice bars popping up that sell good-quality, cold-pressed juices, but homemade is cheaper, and you can be sure of where the produce came from.

HOW TO USE THIS BOOK

Juices do not cure illnesses, but they can contribute physically and psychologically to the process of self-healing. The recipes in this book have been created with specific, common health issues in mind—things my clients regularly come to see me about—but I also want this book to act as a guide to motivate you towards better general health.

The recipes here are good for everyone and can be enjoyed at any time, with food or as a snack. The smoothies can be enjoyed instead of a meal if you have a busy day—it's better to have a smoothie than have nothing to eat and end up starving! You can follow the fast days from time to time and, if you have an ailment, use the recipes specific to your health concern. However, with or without health issues, juices and smoothies are a fantastic way to get a real boost of goodness with minimal effort.

Some drinks are stronger tasting than others, so if you are just starting out, use the recipes that have a higher fruit content, especially berries, and then move onto other ones. You will be surprised how fast you get used to the different tastes. Some of the recipes have unusual ingredients, but most ingredients can be found either in supermarkets or in health food stores.

If there is something you don't like, turn to the Glossary at the back to find alternatives to add instead (page 184). I hope you will grow in confidence and knowledge and learn how to substitute an ingredient for something similar that is easier on your taste buds! Remember that your taste buds will change as you eat less sugar and salt, and include cleaner, more wholesome food in your diet, so you might grow to enjoy ingredients you previously found hard to swallow.

ORGANIC & SEASONAL

I always use organic, if I can, to avoid pesticides. It means that there is no need to peel the produce first (unless using something like a mango, avocado, or papaya), just rinse and you are ready to go. Organic produce can be much more expensive and is not always available, so if this is the case, you might need a little more preparation. For non-organic ingredients, peel what can be peeled and give everything a thorough wash because pesticides are persistent. You'll need to be ultra-careful in your washing, especially with leaves. Lettuce and spinach are among the most contaminated vegetables because they suck up pesticides from the soil and are sprayed the most to prevent the little bugs that love them.

Some ingredients are very seasonal, and if they aren't in season but still on the supermarket shelves, then they may be expensive and it will have taken a lot of air miles to get them there. This is when frozen foods are great. You can get all sorts of organic and non-organic fruits in the freezer section, picked and frozen right away, which preserves their nutrients. Frozen berries or peaches are great in smoothies and juices, and you could also try frozen summer leaves like spinach and spring greens. So you see, there is never an excuse to not eat a rainbow of fruits and vegetables every day!

PREPARATION

I tend not to core anything, but I do remove pits from any fruits that need it. Your juicer and blender will not thank you for putting a plum pit through them. If you use a juicer with a large chute, you shouldn't need to cut anything up. A little tip for juicing small leaves like rosemary is to wrap them in bigger leaves, and pass them through the juicer that way. For smoothies, I core and cube anything that requires it. Peel things like avocados, mangoes, and papaya, basically anything with a tough skin. As I have said, if it is organic you can get away with not peeling, but I would advise you to peel non-organic produce. It is the quickest and easiest way to remove any pesticides that have been used.

For citrus fruits, I prefer to use a citrus press rather than put peeled citrus fruits through the juicer. You can also squeeze the fruit by hand.

EQUIPMENT YOU'LL NEED

For juices   Centrifugal and masticating juicers are easily available on the market, but for the purposes of this book, I used a centrifugal juicer simply because they are more common.

A centrifugal juicer uses a cylindrical grater to spin the juice from the incoming pieces of fruit or vegetables before discarding the pulp. It is fast and super-easy to use. A masticating juicer, on the other hand, creates "cold-pressed" juices by crushing the fruit or vegetables and wringing the juice from the produce. The reason it is COLD pressed is because there is no heat involved, meaning it is raw and the nutrients haven't been damaged by heating. This applies to centrifugal juicing too. You will use smaller quantities of ingredients with a masticating juicer, and it is also an awesome machine when it comes to juicing green leaves. Because it's so efficient, juiced greens will taste stronger. I also prefer juicers with a chute large enough for the produce to be put in whole. There's no point chopping fruit and vegetables when the juicer can do it for you.

For smoothies   I LOVE my NutriBullet because it is so compact and making a smoothie with it is so fast and straightforward. It's amazing, and has such a powerful motor that you can blend everything, skin and all, to a smooth, liquid consistency. It is a drinks blender so it's also smaller than a normal blender, making it good for storage if you don't have much room.

Of course, you can use a normal blender or a hand blender to make smoothies if you have these already. Hand blenders may not cope with raw root vegetables and nuts such as beets and almonds, so go gently and see what you can get away with. If you are going to invest in a blender, make sure that it has a good motor because you don't want to find it burns out the minute you challenge it with a harder piece of fruit or vegetable.

Do a bit of research when you are buying new equipment. For both juicers and smoothies, it is generally better to get one with a higher wattage. This makes a difference in which vegetables and fruits the juicer can cope with. Ideally you do want to be able to juice things like beets and sweet potato easily.

However you make your juice or smoothie, whether it is with a blender or a centrifugal or masticating juicer, you will be making a lovely fruit and vegetable drink and getting all the benefits of their vitamins and minerals.

Now go juice and feel well!

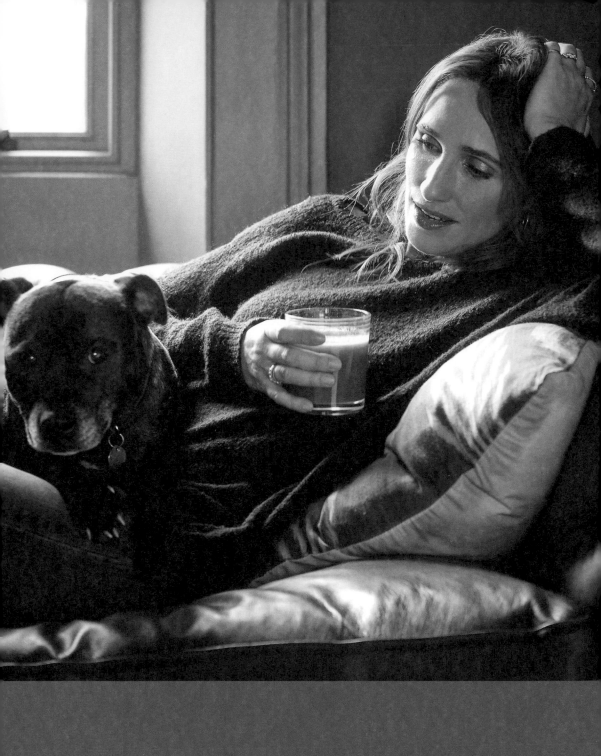

DETOX & HEAL

This chapter is about helping the body's internal system work as well as it can to efficiently eliminate waste and toxins.

In my clinical practice this often means starting with the gut. I find that when the gut is functioning poorly, it can impair a client's health and sense of well-being. The juices included here are all aimed at healing and reinoculating the gut with good bacteria, while calming and soothing any associated pain or bloating.

The liver plays an essential part in ridding the body of toxins, and because we inhabit a world full of stress, pollution, and chemicals, we need to supply it with the nutrition it needs to fight in our corner.

I have included a few hangover juices too—these can be used at any time to aid the liver, not just after a night out . . .

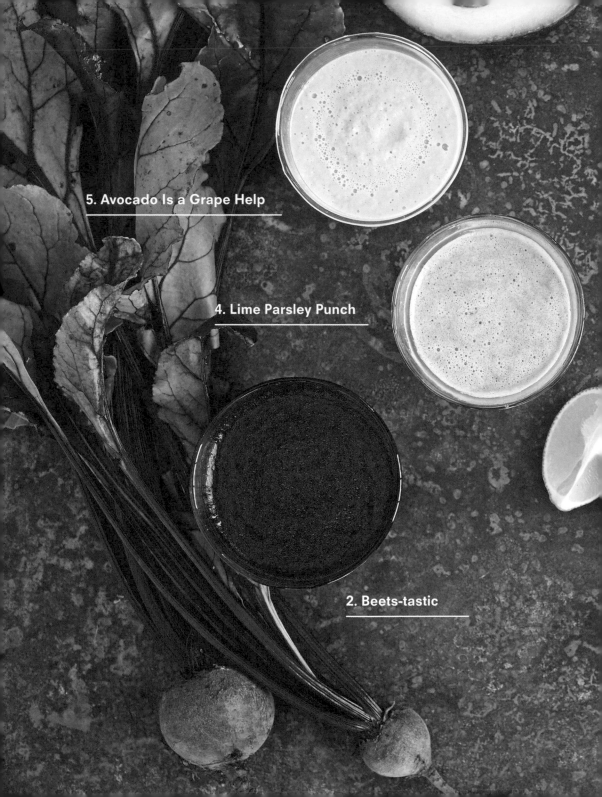

5. Avocado Is a Grape Help

4. Lime Parsley Punch

2. Beets-tastic

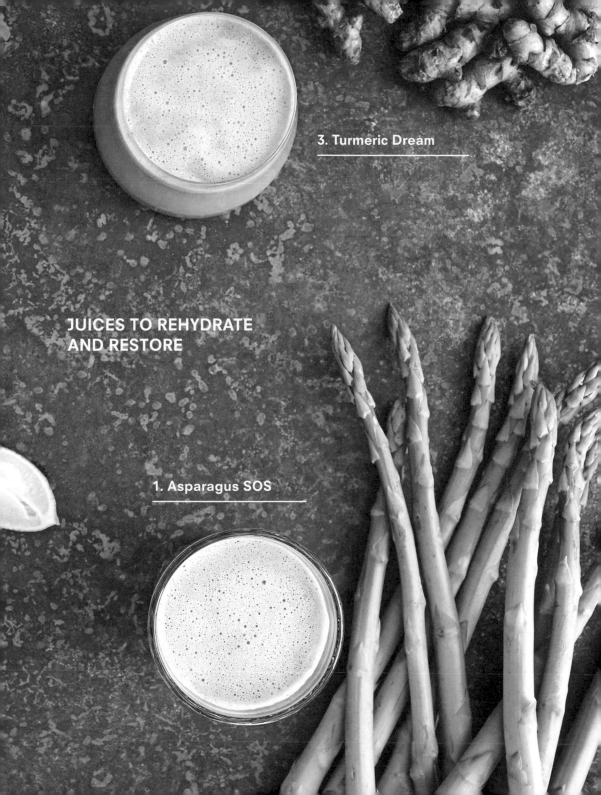

3. Turmeric Dream

JUICES TO REHYDRATE
AND RESTORE

1. Asparagus SOS

1

ASPARAGUS SOS

**small handful of
	spinach**
1 apple
5 spears of asparagus
1 small tomato
**1- to 2-inch piece of
	fresh ginger**
juice of 1 lemon

Asparagus contains enzymes that help break down any alcohol residues left in your system. This amazing juice is packed with antioxidants and is far better than the hair of the dog—any day!

Pass all the ingredients through the juicer, except the lemon juice, stirring it in at the end.

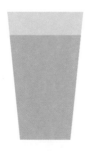

2

BEETS-TASTIC

1 beet
2 stalks of celery
3 handfuls of spinach
juice of ½ lemon
1 tsp spirulina

A body rebalancer for those mornings after the night before . . . This is a blood-cleansing, blood-building, blood-sugar-balancing juice. The spirulina provides protein to help repair any damage in the body.

Pass all the ingredients, except the lemon juice and spirulina, through the juicer. Stir in the lemon juice and spirulina at the end.

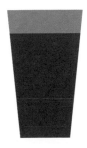

3

TURMERIC DREAM

1 apple
2 carrots
1 stalk of celery
1 pear
juice of 1 lemon
1–2 tsps ground
turmeric (start with
½ tsp and build the
amount up)

This juice will definitely wake you up. The lemon gets the liver going, helping it to produce digestive juices that boost the detox pathways. Turmeric is great for gut health, but it is the curcumin found in turmeric that is the key to this recipe—helping to mop up the acetaldehyde residues left by the alcohol.

Pass all the ingredients, except the lemon juice and turmeric, through the juicer. Stir in the lemon juice and turmeric at the end.

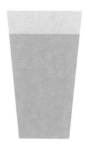

4

LIME PARSLEY PUNCH

1 apple
2 stalks of celery
½ cucumber
1- to 2-inch piece of fresh ginger (you may like to start with less and work up to more)
small handful of parsley
2 handfuls of spinach
juice of ½ lime
juice of ½ lemon

Lime and parsley pack a punch. The sharpness in the taste is tempered by the sweetness of the apple. It is a great alkalizing juice, while the cucumber and parsley act as a gentle diuretic that can help to eliminate more toxins. Ginger is great if you're also feeling a little woozy . . .

Pass all the ingredients through the juicer, except the lime and lemon juice, stirring them in at the end.

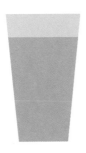

5

AVOCADO IS A GRAPE HELP (SMOOTHIE)

2 apples
½ avocado, pitted and
**   peeled**
15 grapes
handful of spinach
2 stalks of celery
juice of 1 lime
1–2 cups (250–500 ml)
**   filtered water**

This smoothie will get you out the door. Blood sugar is often a problem after a night out, which is why we tend to opt for a sugary snack. This smoothie is a more substantial solution because of its natural sugars and fats. The avocado is in a class of its own. It has an unusually high number of benefits, including good fats to help your body recover. With all the antioxidants that are in spinach and lime, along with the resveratrol in the grapes, you'll be feeling as fresh as a daisy!

Chop the apples, avocado, grapes, spinach and celery into manageable sizes for your blender. Add the lime juice to the blender and whiz it up along with all the other ingredients.

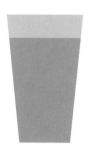

6

GREEN CLEANSE

1 peach, pitted
½ cucumber
2 handfuls of any kale
handful of Swiss chard
juice of ½ lemon
juice of 1 lime

Green Cleanse will definitely give the liver a boost. It is a dark green juice with a high concentration of cruciferous vegetables. These vegetables provide your liver with the nutrients it needs to start detoxing.

Pass all the ingredients through the juicer, except the lemon and lime juice, stirring them in at the end.

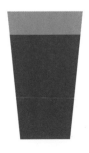

6. Green Cleanse

9. Daily Helper

DETOX FROM THE INSIDE, STARTING WITH THE LIVER

10. Not for the Faint Hearted

8. Liver Cleanse

7. Super Green

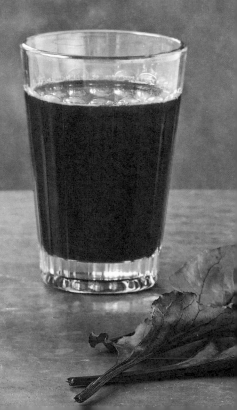
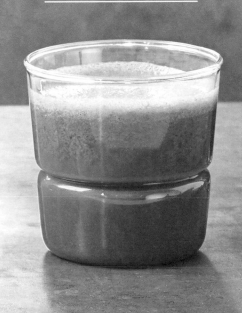

7

SUPER GREEN

2 lacinato kale leaves
handful of spinach
handful of kale
2 stalks of celery
small handful of
    parsley
1 apple
½ pear
8 raspberries
juice of 1 lime

This juice is amazingly nutrient dense. It is a powerhouse of antioxidants and sulfur-containing vegetables, all geared up to assist the liver and the production of glutathione, which is THE most essential antioxidant in the body!

Pass all the ingredients through the juicer, except the lemon juice, stirring it in at the end.

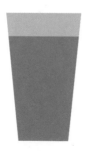

8

LIVER CLEANSE

½ **globe artichoke**
3 **beet leaves**
1 **beet**
¼ **cucumber**
1 **stalk of celery**
1 **apple**
1- **to 2-inch piece of**
   fresh ginger
juice of ½ lemon

The liver is essential to our feeling of well-being and is where a lot of the hard work of toxin removal happens. If it is under par we feel sluggish— so best to give it some love! Beet and beet greens are excellent blood cleansers, while artichoke contains the flavonoid silymarin (the active ingredient in milk thistle), which is protective of the liver. It's no surprise then that a juice with a lot of beet and artichoke is very supportive to our lovely liver.

Remove the stalk and the tougher outer leaves of the artichoke and juice the rest. Pass all the ingredients through the juicer, except the lemon juice, stirring it in at the end.

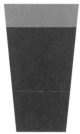

9

DAILY HELPER

1 apple
1 carrot
1 beetroot
handful of watercress
10 raspberries
   (optional)
milk thistle extract
   (as directed on the
   bottle)

This is a classic juice with a little twist, and a great everyday juice to keep the antioxidants up and the toxins down. Milk thistle is a wonderful herb that is well known for its liver protective properties. Combined with watercress—a bitter herb that gets the bile juices going—and the huge antioxidant power of carrot and beet, you'll be absolutely on top of the world!

Pass all the ingredients, except for the milk thistle, through the juicer. Add the milk thistle drops at the end after the juicing is complete, following the directions on the bottle.

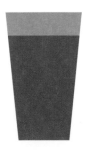

10

NOT FOR THE FAINT HEARTED

handful of parsley
3 spears of asparagus
3 dandelion leaves
1 clove of garlic
juice of 2 lemons
juice of 2 oranges

This little number will give you a real lift! It's an intense juice, but really worth it. I love it—the garlic, lemon, and parsley—what's not to love? It's a sulfur-rich juice, which the liver needs in order to function optimally. Added to this are the protective qualities to the liver of asparagus and dandelion. This juice is just a complete liver before-and-after care package.

Pass all the ingredients through the juicer, except the lemon and orange juice. You can either juice the garlic or crush it and stir in. Juicing it can leave your juicer with a garlicky taste for a few juices, which I don't mind, but you might! Crushing it will mean you get more garlic, as a lot can get stuck in a juicer, depending on which type you are using. Stir in the lemon and orange juice at the end.

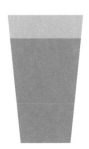

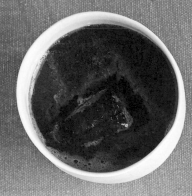

15. Fire in the Belly

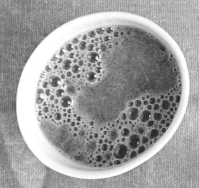

12. A Bit of Papaya

11. Tummy Help

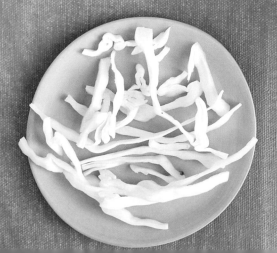

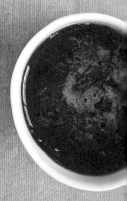

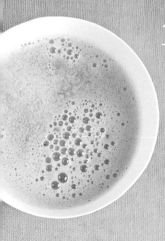

13. Bloat Away! ————————

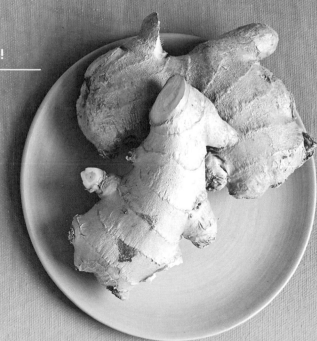

HEAL YOUR GUT

14. Calm Yourself ————

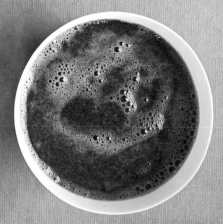

11

TUMMY HELP

¼ **pineapple, peeled**
¼ **red or white cabbage**
1 beet
2 carrots
2 handfuls of spinach
juice of ½ orange
juice of ½ lemon

This is an amazing juice for inflammation in the gut. It soothes and calms the tummy. Cabbage is very healing as it contains the essential amino acid, glutamine. The betacyanin in beets is protective and helps normal cell function. Pineapple contains bromelain, which is a powerful anti-inflammatory, and also contains enzymes that promote digestion.

Chop the cabbage into manageable pieces for your juicer. Pass all the ingredients through the juicer, except the orange and lemon juice, stirring them in at the end.

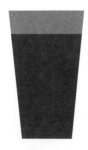

12

A BIT OF PAPAYA

½ small papaya, peeled
handful of kale
handful of cabbage
2-inch piece of fresh
    ginger
squeeze of lemon juice
juice of ½ lime

This juice comes to the rescue of many ailments related to the gut. The papain in papaya is a fantastic digestive enzyme, which is helpful for your digestion. Ginger, which is one of my favorite spices, in this recipe can help reduce gas and feelings of nausea. Cabbage is an excellent source of the essential amino acid, glutamine, which will help to heal the gut and is GREAT for ulcers.

Pass all the ingredients through the juicer, except the lemon and lime juice, stirring them in at the end.

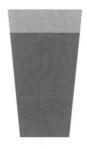

13

BLOAT AWAY!

½ small pineapple, rind removed
½ fennel bulb
2 stalks of celery
2- to 4-inch piece of fresh ginger (you may need to work up to higher amounts of ginger—it can be quite strong)

That's right! Bloat away! Bloating is a real problem for many people and can be extremely uncomfortable. The ingredients in this juice can really help. Pineapple has helpful digestive enzymes, but the secret to this juice is the fennel and ginger. They combine to build up good prebiotic gut bacteria, which helps the gut deal with food more efficiently, and therefore reduces bloating.

Pass all the ingredients through the juicer.

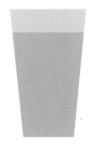

14

CALM YOURSELF

½ cucumber
2 stalks of celery
¼ fennel bulb
handful of mint leaves
1- to 2-inch piece of
**   fresh ginger**
1 apple
10 blueberries
juice of 1 lime (optional)

The fennel and mint in this juice make it very soothing to a gut caught in spasm. Mint is also understood to be helpful with IBS due to its calming qualities, helping the muscles in the gut to relax. It is also a good juice if water retention is causing bloating. The cucumber and celery will help to relieve this because of their diuretic action, and they are also great for hydration because of their high water content.

Pass all the ingredients through the juicer, except the lemon juice if using, stirring it in at the end.

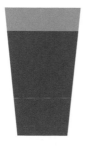

15

FIRE IN THE BELLY

¼ small cabbage
1 apple
1 stalk of celery
1- to 2-inch piece of
fresh ginger
15 red grapes
1 lemon, with peel
1 tsp apple cider
vinegar

This is an amazing juice for the fire in your belly. Most people suffering from reflux or indigestion are actually prone to LOW stomach acid. Here we have a juice that is super alkalizing to the body tissue, while the apple cider vinegar helps our stomach acid and digestive juices get going and therefore aids digestion.

Chop the cabbage into manageable pieces for your juicer. Pass all the ingredients, except the vinegar, through the juicer, including the whole lemon with its peel. Stir in the apple cider vinegar after you have made the main juice.

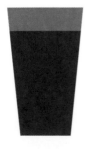

16

GET MOVING (SMOOTHIE)

½ papaya, peeled
½ banana, peeled
½ apple
1 tbsp sunflower seeds
1 tbsp ground
    flaxseeds
1 tbsp aloe vera juice
1–2 cups (250–500 ml)
    filtered water
2 tsps mixed green
    powder (a mix
    of spirulina,
    wheatgrass,
    chlorella, etc.)

This is a fantastic smoothie to get things moving if they've become slightly blocked . . . ! Once a day is the minimum we want to be going to the loo, so using this smoothie will keep you nice and regular. Your bowel will appreciate it—the smoothie is very alkalizing, which keeps the colon happy, and this will mean a happier and more vital you.

Blend all the ingredients together, except the green powder, stirring it in at the end.

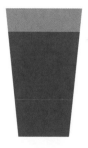

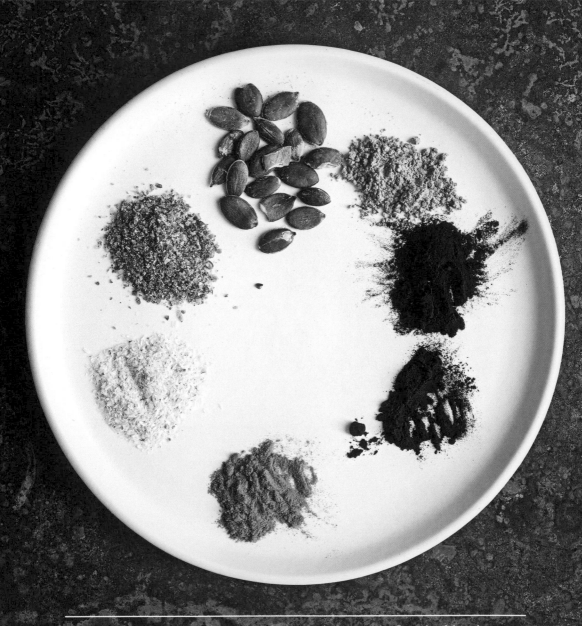

Good for the Gut (clockwise from top): Pumpkin Seeds, Matcha Green Tea Powder, Spirulina, Chlorella Powder, Turmeric, Psyllium Husks, Ground Flaxseeds

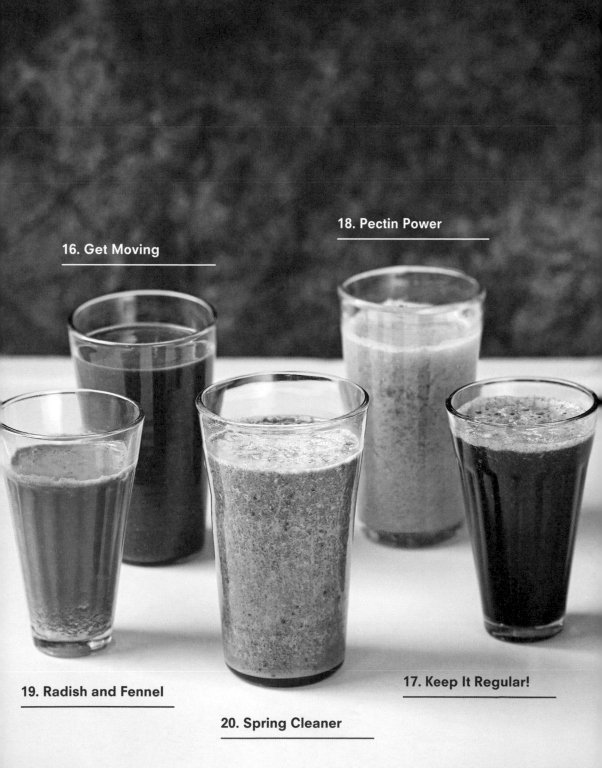

18. Pectin Power

16. Get Moving

19. Radish and Fennel

20. Spring Cleaner

17. Keep It Regular!

17

KEEP IT REGULAR!

**10 blackberries
2 pears
1 head of romaine
    lettuce
2 tsps mixed green
    powder (a mix
    of spirulina,
    wheatgrass,
    chlorella, etc.)**

With a high water content from the lettuce, this juice should help hydrate the body and therefore the stools, making it easier for a bowel movement and to keep everything moving. As well as tasting yummy, the blackberries and pears have a good amount of soluble fiber to help cleanse the bowel.

Juice the fruit and lettuce, and then add the green powder, stirring it in at the end.

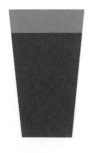

18

PECTIN POWER

1 peach, pitted
¼ Savoy cabbage
1 apple
1 carrot
1 fig (if you suffer from
**   IBS, leave out the fig)**
small handful of
**   kohlrabi**

Pectin is a soluble fiber, and is present in each of the ingredients in this juice. Figs soothe the intestines, are high in minerals, and are also alkalizing to the body. Cabbage is high in glutamine, which is healing to the gut. Everything about this juice makes it lovely for any day. Add ginger for a little bit of extra heat.

Chop the cabbage into manageable pieces for your juicer, then pass all the ingredients through the juicer.

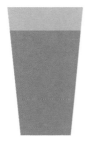

19

RADISH AND FENNEL

5 radishes
¼ fennel bulb
1 sweet potato
**1- to 2-inch piece of
   fresh ginger**
1 clove of garlic
juice of 2 lemons
juice of 1 orange

High in prebiotic foods, this concentrated juice helps to reinoculate the gut with good bacteria, while the garlic will help to remove any unwanted bacteria. These good bacteria help the smooth running of the gut and the breakdown and elimination of toxins from the body. You will notice the difference if the colony in your gut is in balance—so be brave and reward your gut with this powerful juice.

Pass all the ingredients through the juicer, except the lemon and orange juice. You can either juice the garlic or crush it and stir in. Juicing it can leave your juicer with a garlicky taste for a few juices, which I don't mind, but you might! Crushing it will mean you get more garlic, as a lot can get stuck in a juicer, depending on which type you are using. Stir in the lemon and orange juice at the end.

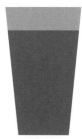

20

SPRING CLEANER (SMOOTHIE)

4 dandelion leaves
10 blueberries
1 tsp ground turmeric
1 tbsp flaxseed oil
1 tsp psyllium husks
2 cups (500 ml) filtered
**   water**
juice of 1 lemon

Psyllium husk acts as a loofah to the colon, cleaning as it moves through the digestive system. Dandelion is very beneficial if you're trying to detox, while the flaxseed oil coats the digestive system and helps easy transit. The turmeric will help reduce any inflammation.

Add all the ingredients to a blender and whiz together.

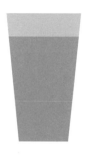

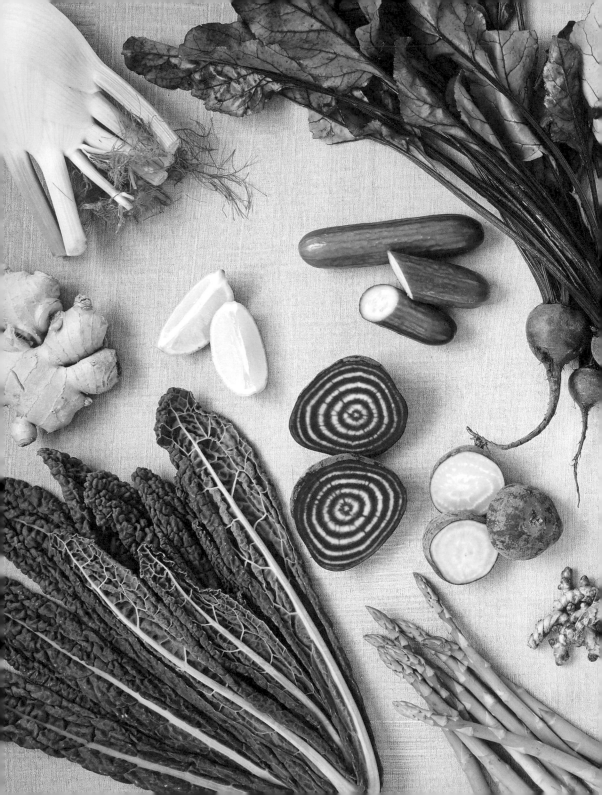

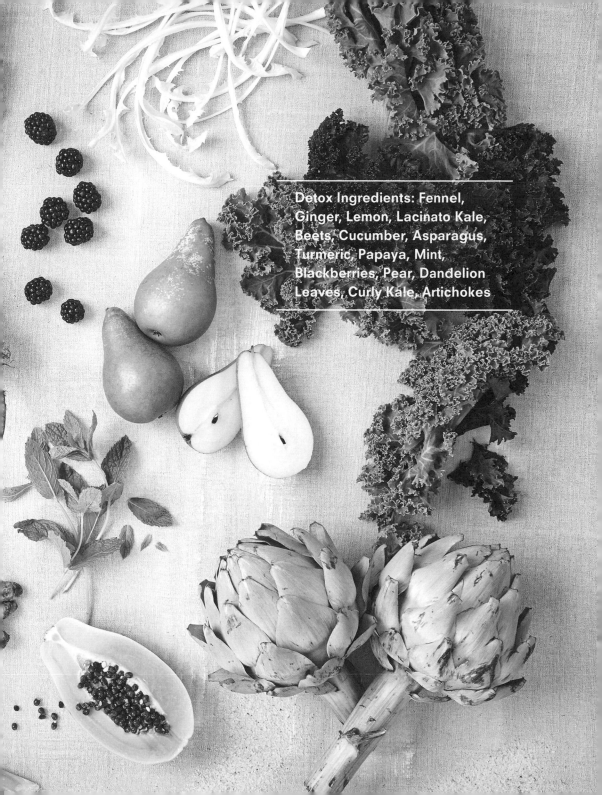

Detox Ingredients: Fennel, Ginger, Lemon, Lacinato Kale, Beets, Cucumber, Asparagus, Turmeric, Papaya, Mint, Blackberries, Pear, Dandelion Leaves, Curly Kale, Artichokes

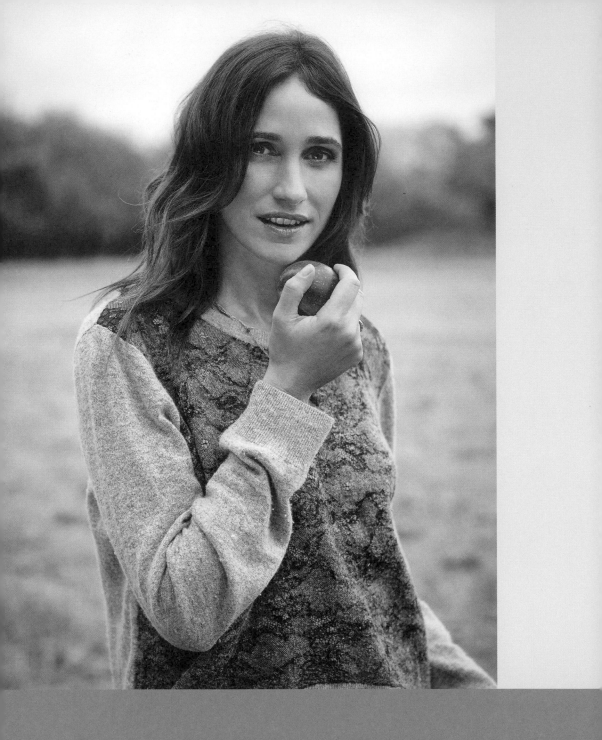

REST
& DE-STRESS

Everyday life can be very hectic. Consequently, we rarely allow ourselves to switch off completely and the adrenal glands that deal with stress hormones can become worn out, leaving us feeling energy-less, exhausted, and ultimately pretty miserable. The juices in this chapter are here to lend a helping hand.

A myriad of causes contribute to making us feel low, but if you experience loss of sleep, or feel down or anxious, you may be unwittingly adding to the self-neglect.

Taking small steps to effect big changes will ultimately make a positive difference to your outlook. Something as simple as having a juice can help get you back on track. The ingredients used in these juices are high in B vitamins and minerals, such as magnesium and the amino acid tryptophan, which in combination are geared toward helping the body cope with stress, and to relax and enhance a more affirmative mood.

Lower stress and being more relaxed will release a "yippee" feeling, and lead to more serene sleep.

RELAX AND UNWIND

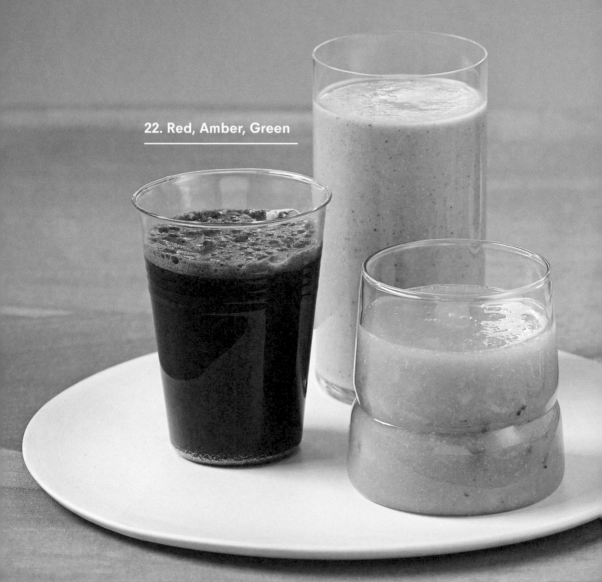

21. Chill

22. Red, Amber, Green

24. LMC

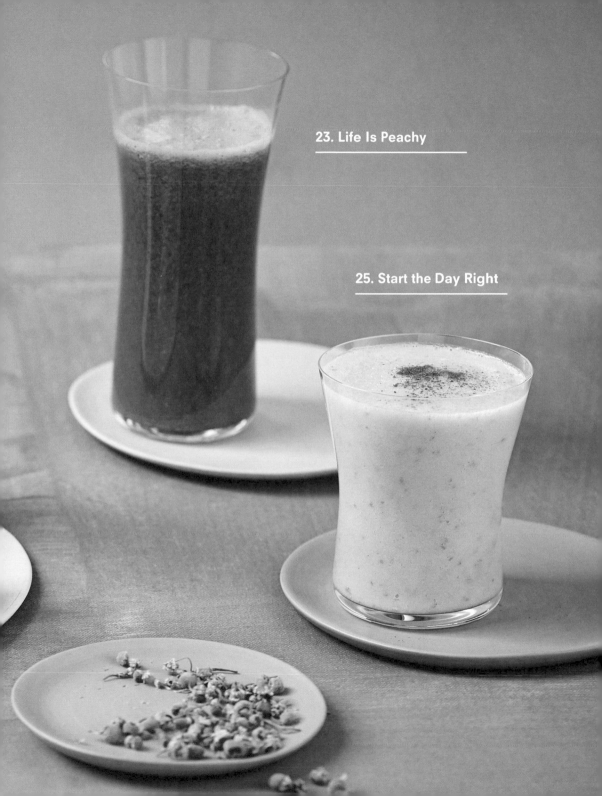

23. Life Is Peachy

25. Start the Day Right

21

CHILL (SMOOTHIE)

1 cup (250 ml) iced
   chamomile tea
1 banana, peeled
1 pear
1 cup (250 ml)
   unsweetened
   almond milk or
   filtered water
2 tsps maca powder
1 tbsp pumpkin seeds

The nutrients in this smoothie will surely help you to relax. The other ingredient that helps you to de-stress is the high level of the amino acid tyrosine, which is super helpful if your adrenals are exhausted and you're finding life all a bit much. The iced chamomile tea is a lovely thing to have in the fridge if you want to make extra!

To make the iced chamomile tea, make the tea as you normally would, then leave it to infuse for 5 minutes at least. You can then leave it to cool or add ice to it if you want to cool it fast. Place all the ingredients in the blender and give them a whiz.

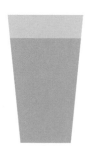

22

RED, AMBER, GREEN

½ sweet potato
3 leaves of spring
  greens
handful of parsley
1 red pepper
2 carrots
2-inch piece of fresh
  ginger

This juice is high in B vitamins, which help the nervous system remain calm. It is also high in vitamins C and A, which help rid the body of free radicals caused by stress. This juice really nourishes, and allows you to cope more successfully with stress. It is a potent nutrient vehicle.

I don't peel the sweet potato, but you can if you prefer, then pass all the ingredients through the juicer.

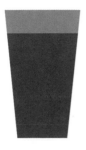

23

LIFE IS PEACHY

2 peaches, pitted
2 handfuls of spinach
**   or Swiss chard**
1 zucchini

I love peaches. When they are in season they are a fantastic fruit to use. High in antioxidants, selenium, lycopene, and lutein, they are a superb supporter of the cardiovascular system, which suffers when we're stressed out. The spinach or chard is the magnesium factor here, and will help you chill. Combined with the zucchini, they make this juice high in soluble fiber, which will help clear stress hormones from the body.

Pass everything through the juicer.

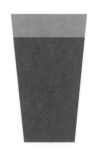

24

LMC (LACINATO KALE, MANGO, AND CARROT)

1 mango, peeled and pitted
handful of lacinato kale
1 carrot
juice of 1 lemon

When we are stressed, our digestion can be impaired because the brain is focusing on other matters. The mango in this juice will help you out with its digestive enzymes. This juice is hydrating, and high in antioxidants and contains B vitamins, so it's a good juice for your digestion when you are in a stressed condition.

Pass all the ingredients through the juicer, except the lemon juice, stirring it in at the end.

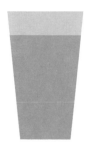

25

START THE DAY RIGHT (SMOOTHIE)

1½ tsps soaked and
   drained oats
1–2 cups (250–500
   ml) unsweetened
   almond milk or
   filtered water
handful of kohlrabi
   leaves or whatever
   green leaves you
   have
1 apple
1 tsp ground cinnamon
2-inch piece of fresh
   ginger

Oats are a great source of B vitamins, which we need for our nervous system to run smoothly. Oats are also extremely soothing to the gut. With the oats and almond milk being high in magnesium, this makes for a very comforting smoothie. It will keep you on an even keel and is a great start to the day, as it produces a slow, steady release of energy.

Soak the oats before you make the smoothie for at least 30 minutes or overnight (see page 187), then add all the ingredients to your blender and off you go. You can grate the ginger in if you prefer.

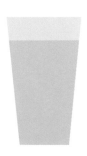

26

HAPPY EVERY DAY (SMOOTHIE)

1 banana, peeled
1 zucchini
10 raspberries
2 tsps pumpkin seeds
1 tsp maca powder
1 cup (150 g) ice cubes
½ cup (125 ml) filtered
    water

This smoothie is high in tryptophan, which is essential to make serotonin, a good-mood chemical that stimulates both happiness and sleep. Maca helps to fight fatigue, and if you aren't tired but full of energy, it will sustain energy levels—yippee!

Place all the ingredients into a blender and whiz together.

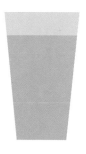

BOOST YOUR MOOD

29. Not So Bleak Midwinter

26. Happy Every Day

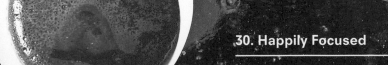

30. Happily Focused

27. Feeling Good, Feeling Fine
_____

28. Smiley Happy People
_____

27

FEELING GOOD, FEELING FINE

handful of spinach
¼ head of broccoli
½ sweet potato
1 red pepper
juice of 2 oranges

Get some oxygen circulating inside you to feel more vital and well. These vegetables contain great amounts of iron, needed to transport oxygen around the body. More oxygen means more energy—you'll feel on top of the world!

If you have hypothyroidism, steam the broccoli before you juice it or replace with spinach or Swiss chard.

Pass all the ingredients through the juicer, except the orange juice, stirring it in at the end.

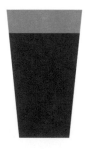

28

SMILEY HAPPY PEOPLE

handful of Swiss chard
handful of lacinato kale
2 apples
10 blueberries
5 strawberries

Simply drinking this juice will cheer you up. It is high in folate (vitamin B9), which is thought to help relieve symptoms of depression. The berries and apples are high in phytonutrients, which assist the levels of serotonin and dopamine. If these can become a regular feature in your diet, they should help your mood to stay positive.

Pass all the ingredients through the juicer.

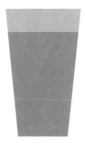

29

NOT SO BLEAK MIDWINTER

1 apple
1 carrot
½ sweet potato
**2-inch piece of fresh
    ginger**
juice of 1 lemon
½ tsp raw honey

A warming and cozy juice. The raw honey is antibacterial, antiviral, and delicious too. It should lift your mood and help you stay in good health throughout the winter. A juice to keep you feeling well and put a spring in your step.

Pass all the ingredients through the juicer, except the lemon juice and honey, stirring them in at the end. You could add ground cinnamon to this too.

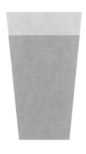

30

HAPPILY FOCUSED

1 carrot
½ sweet potato
1 nectarine, pitted
juice of 1 orange
1 tsp ground cinnamon
1 tbsp flaxseed oil

Great if you're suffering from dreaded brain fog. This juice is rich in folic acid, which is helpful for good brain function and concentration. It is also high in beta-carotene and magnesium from the carrot and nectarine, which will help you relax. I have added flaxseed oil because our brains need essential fatty acids to work well, so stir in the omegas!

Pass the vegetables and fruit through the juicer. Stir the orange juice, cinnamon, and flaxseed oil into the finished juice.

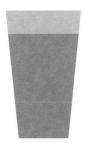

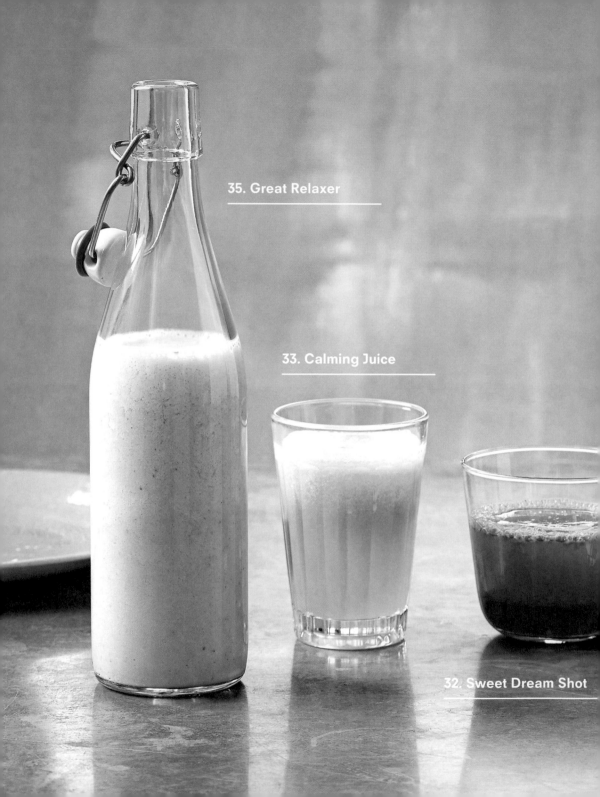

35. Great Relaxer

33. Calming Juice

32. Sweet Dream Shot

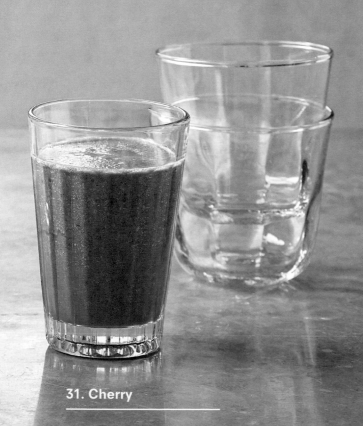

SLEEP WELL, REST EASY

34. Muscle Relaxant

31. Cherry

31

CHERRY (SMOOTHIE)

2 cups (500 ml) iced chamomile tea
15 fresh or frozen sour cherries, pitted (if you can't find sour cherries, use normal cherries)
½ banana, peeled
5 almonds

Bananas, cherries, and almonds are all high in tryptophan. This is what our body needs to make serotonin, which is converted into melatonin, our sleep hormone. If pitting the cherries hasn't made you tired already, then this will help you have a lovely sleep.

To make the iced chamomile tea, make the tea as you normally would, then leave it to infuse for 5 minutes at least. You can then leave it to cool or add ice to it if you want to cool it fast. Then blend all the ingredients together for a lovely smoothie.

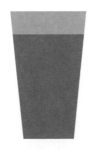

32

SWEET DREAM SHOT

juice of 1–2 oranges
juice of 1 lemon
a shot of wheatgrass,
**   or 2 tsps wheatgrass**
powder

Wheatgrass is healing to the body, and the citrus in this concentrated juice contains inositol, which is thought to calm anxiety and enhance sleep. It is low in liquids too, so you won't be up all night going to the bathroom! Sweet dreams!

Mix all the ingredients together in a glass and give it a stir.

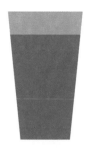

33

CALMING JUICE

¼ **honeydew melon,**
   rind removed
handful of kale
3 lemon balm leaves
   (do not use
   if you have
   hypothyroidism)

Kale is high in pretty much everything, but we need its B vitamins and magnesium. B vitamins are essential to keeping the nervous system working well, and keeping anxiety to a minimum. Lemon balm is a relative of the mint family and is believed to reduce stress and promote sleep.

Pass all the ingredients through a juicer.

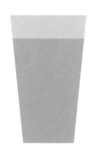

34

MUSCLE RELAXANT (SMOOTHIE)

1 banana, peeled
handful of spinach
7 almonds
2 cups (500 ml)
    coconut water

Each element in this smoothie contains magnesium and potassium, so any tension you might be feeling in your muscles should easily melt away.

Place all the ingredients in a blender and whiz together.

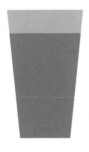

35

GREAT RELAXER (SMOOTHIE)

1 banana, peeled
1 cup (250 ml)
  unsweetened
  almond milk
5 almonds
1 tsp ground cinnamon
  (optional)

This smoothie should relax you. Full of magnesium and tryptophan, it will help you get a good night's sleep.

Blend all the ingredients together.

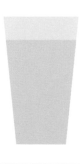

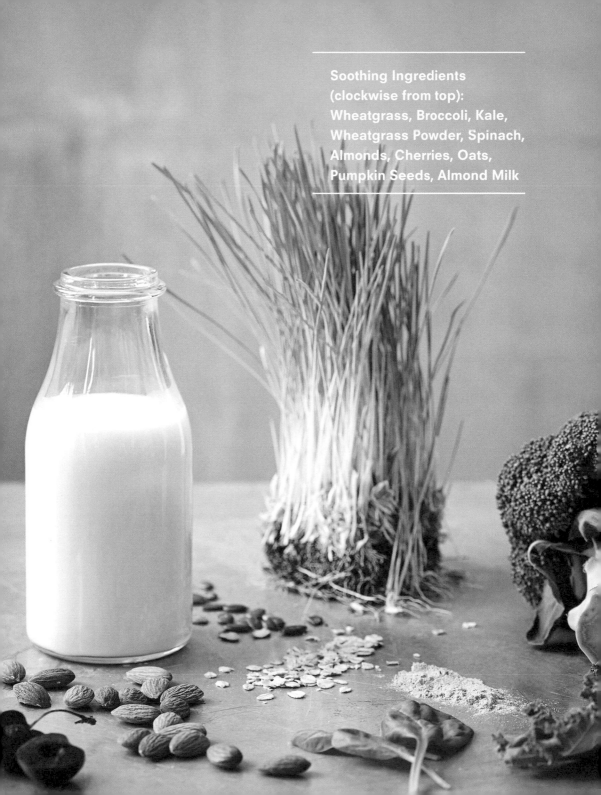

Soothing Ingredients
(clockwise from top):
Wheatgrass, Broccoli, Kale,
Wheatgrass Powder, Spinach,
Almonds, Cherries, Oats,
Pumpkin Seeds, Almond Milk

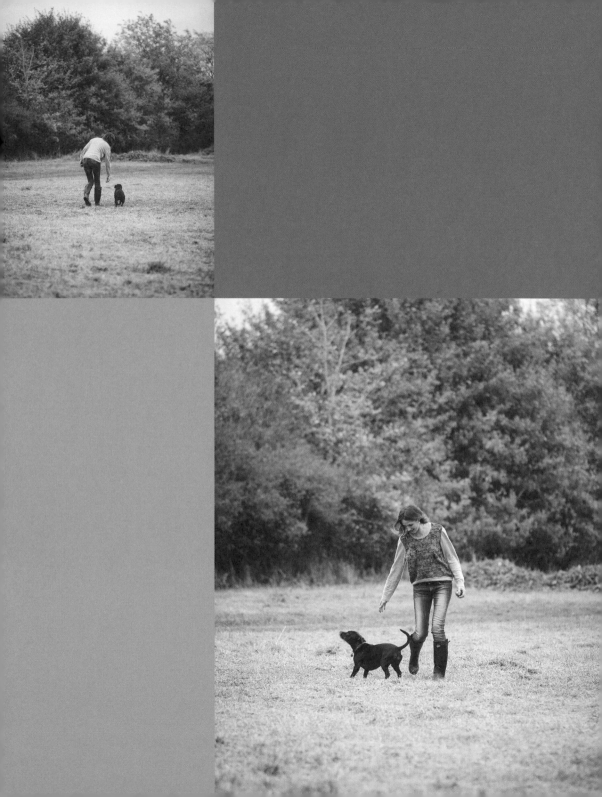

ENERGIZE

Exhausted . . . that's what I hear people say all the time. It's easy to blame exhaustion solely on a busy schedule, but it always makes me wonder what fuel people are putting into their bodies. We are such amazing, complicated biological machines, and we work best when we have the necessary supply of nutrients supporting our system.

These juices will help to balance your blood sugar levels and leave you feeling much more energized throughout the whole day, without that mid-afternoon slump or mood swings.

Our intake of sugar and processed food is out of control and can contribute to many problems, including diabetes and heart problems. Juices are nutrition power-houses and are a great way of getting extra nutrients into your system (on top of your perfect nutrient-dense vegan diet, obviously!). Taking in more fruit and vegetables helps to alkalize our body, which becomes very acidic when we are eating and drinking modern-day foods.

You can use these juices and smoothies anytime, and if you start having one instead of a naughty mid-afternoon snack, you will not only feel very virtuous, but also lighter and more energetic for the rest of the day.

BOOST YOUR ENERGY LEVELS

37. Marvelous Maca

40. Wheatgrass Power

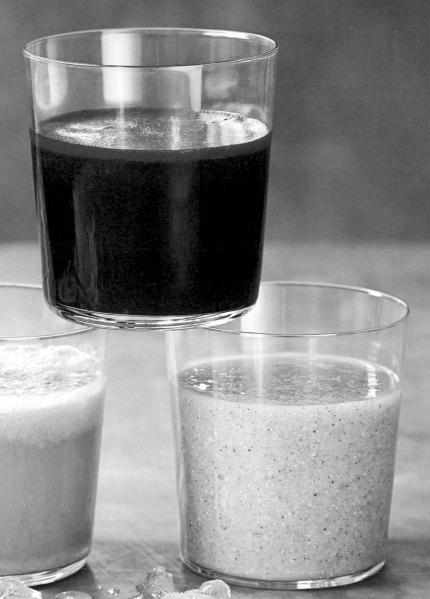

36. Crystal Clear

38. Apple and Carrot with a Twist

39. Sprouting with Energy

36

CRYSTAL CLEAR

¼ pineapple, rind removed
2 beets
2 stalks of celery
6 radishes
1 tsp rosemary leaves
1 tsp thyme leaves
6 sage leaves

Rosemary is well known for helping your memory and concentration. The sage will help balance your hormones, especially if you are at the start of menopause, as it can really help with hot flashes. The combination of these herbs will help the brain fog clear, and leave you feeling like you can take on the world!

Pass all the ingredients through the juicer, wrapping the rosemary and thyme into the sage leaves, otherwise they will get lost in the juicer.

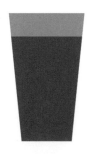

37

MARVELOUS MACA

1 carrot
1 cucumber
juice of 1 lemon
2 tsps maca powder
½–1 tsp cayenne
pepper

Marvelous maca powder has two groups of unique compounds called macamides and macaenes that are thought to be great at boosting energy levels. Its high iron content helps oxygen levels in the blood, which in turn helps us feel brighter and more energetic.

Pass the carrot and cucumber through the juicer. Stir in the lemon juice, maca powder, and cayenne pepper.

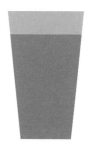

38

APPLE AND CARROT WITH A TWIST

2 apples
3 carrots
2 handfuls of parsley
4- to 6-inch piece of
    fresh ginger
    (start small as this
    is a lot of ginger and
    may be too strong
    for you)
juice of 1 lemon

This juice is one of the first ones I ever had. It is such a good staple and delivers a huge range of phytonutrients. I have tailored it very slightly to help energy levels by simply adding parsley, ginger, and lemon. Parsley is full of chlorophyll and is understood to assist energy levels.

Juice all the ingredients together, except the lemon juice, stirring it in at the end.

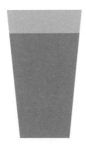

39

SPROUTING WITH ENERGY (SMOOTHIE)

**2 kiwifruits, peeled
1 apple
juice of 1 lime
¼ cucumber
2 tsps chia seeds
handful of sprouted
   alfalfa seeds or any
   sprouts (mung, lentil,
   sunflower, etc.)
1 cup (250 ml)
   filtered water
½ cup (75 g) ice cubes**

So let's talk sprouts . . . sprouts are packed full of protein, vitamins, minerals, and enzymes and are bursting with energy. Think about how much energy they require to grow—it's what we want and what we get from using sprouted seeds and sprouted legumes in smoothies. This smoothie is another way of rehydrating and is a particularly nutrient-dense drink.

Add all the ingredients to your blender and whiz up.

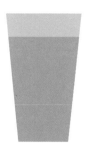

40

WHEATGRASS POWER

¼ pineapple, rind
   removed
2 apricots, pitted
1 cup (150 g)
   blackberries
1 pear
handful of mint leaves
a shot of wheatgrass or
   2 tsps wheatgrass
   powder

High in antioxidants and very lovely to the taste buds, this juice will give you a boost. The wheatgrass is high in chlorophyll and abundant in vitamins, which help the body's energy levels by boosting the body's metabolism. You should feel pretty up for anything after this one!

Juice everything together. If you are using a masticating cold press juicer, you will be able to make a wheatgrass shot while making this juice, otherwise stir in the wheatgrass powder at the end.

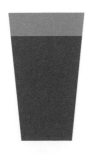

41

SWEET AND SAFE

2 pears
1 apple
15 blueberries
2 tsps ground cinnamon

Yes, this juice is packed full of fruit and yes, fruit is high in natural sugars, but what we also have here is a combination high in soluble fiber, which slows the absorption of sugar into the body. This juice also has a high content of chromium, which can be useful for the efficient use of insulin in the body. The cinnamon is a natural blood-sugar-balancing friend. All in all, it should suit a sweet tooth, while helping to balance energy-release in the body.

Juice all the ingredients together, except the cinnamon, stirring it in at the end.

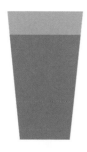

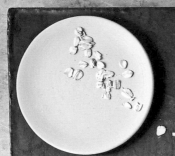

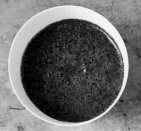

48. On an Even Kale

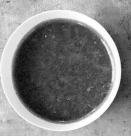

47. Beyond Balanced

42. Chromium Balance

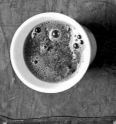

44. Visionary

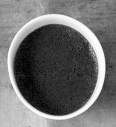

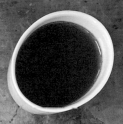

46. Balanced

43. Just Dreamy

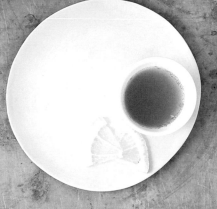

49. Good Morning . . . Good Day

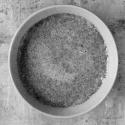

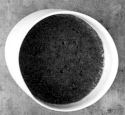

41. Sweet and Safe

45. Blueberries and Other Things

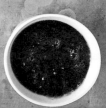

50. Feeling Candy

42

CHROMIUM BALANCE

4 spears of asparagus
¼ head of broccoli
1 sweet potato
10 red grapes

Insulin is the hormone that helps our body process sugars, and since we live in such a sweet (sugary) world, we need all the help we can get to keep our insulin working at an optimum. Foods rich in chromium have been used for years to help balance blood sugar. This juice contains vegetables and fruit that are high in this gem, and will help stave off fatigue, stress, and any blood sugar problems.

If you suffer from hypothyroidism, steam the broccoli before you juice it, or substitute for 6 green beans or a carrot.

Juice all the ingredients together.

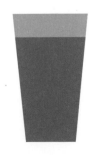

43

JUST DREAMY

¼ small watermelon, rind removed

1 apple (green if you are diabetic)

10 blueberries

juice of 1 lemon

1 tsp ground turmeric

1 tsp ground cinnamon

This is sooooo delicious! I often speak to clients who seem to have forgotten how delicious fruit is. This juice will remind anyone who has forgotten about the fabulousness of fresh, natural, clean food. Besides the just dreamy taste, it actually benefits the body in many ways that are important if you're diabetic—it alkalizes the body, which is important for all of us, and helps balance blood sugar levels, and therefore energy levels, throughout the day.

Juice the watermelon with the apple and blueberries. Stir in the lemon juice, turmeric, and cinnamon at the end.

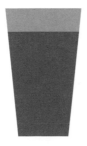

44

VISIONARY

5 green beans
¼ head of broccoli
10 raspberries
5 strawberries
2 carrots

This is a wonderful juice and is good for us at any time, though the ingredients in it are specifically aimed at helping your eyes to stay healthy. These fruits and veggies are thought to help reduce the risk of macular degeneration, which you are at a greater risk from if you are diabetic.

If you have hypothyroidism, steam the broccoli before you juice it or replace with spinach or Swiss chard.

Juice all the ingredients together.

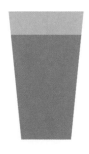

45

BLUEBERRIES AND OTHER THINGS

20 blueberries
½ cucumber
2-inch piece of fresh ginger (start with a small amount as it can be quite strong)
juice of ½ lemon

This juice is good for blood sugar balancing and insulin resistance. It has a lot of chromium in it, and the cucumber will help hydration, while the lemon gives it an alkalizing zing!

Pass all the ingredients through the juicer, except the lemon juice, stirring it in at the end.

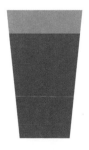

46

BALANCED (SMOOTHIE)

¼ cup (25g) soaked
   and drained oats
Seeds from ½
   pomegranate
½ apple
½ beet
2 spears of asparagus
2 cups (500 ml)
   filtered water
1 tbsp flaxseed oil

A strong-tasting smoothie, but loaded with nutrition for blood sugar control. This smoothie will help support your body and its use of insulin. Pomegranate gives the smoothie loads of antioxidant power.

Soak the oats before you make the smoothie for at least 30 minutes or overnight (see page 187). Put the soaked oats in the blender with all the other ingredients and blend together.

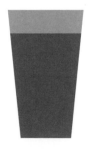

47

BEYOND BALANCED (SMOOTHIE)

¼ **watermelon, rind removed**
small handful of sprouted sunflower seeds (or something similar)
1 cup (150 g) frozen blueberries or raspberries
handful of spinach
1 tsp maca powder
1 tsp chlorella powder

High in chromium, this smoothie will help your energy levels stay constant rather than peaking and dipping, leaving you exhausted. The maca is supportive for depleted adrenal glands, which struggle if you're up and down all day. It is also high in other blood-sugar-friendly nutrients that help to keep you on the level.

Put all the ingredients in the blender and blend together.

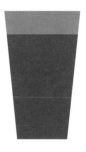

48

ON AN EVEN KALE

4 kale leaves
1 apple (green if you
    are diabetic)
1 small pear
1 tsp spirulina
2 tsps ground
    cinnamon (build up
    to this amount, start
    small!)

This is a boosting juice that helps if you're feeling fatigued in the morning. Much better than reaching for sugary drinks or food. It's a superb versatile juice, a great way to start the day—in fact, a great way to start every day! It contains soluble fiber, which slows the absorption of fruit sugars into the body. Because the absorption process is slower, we get more chance to take in the nutrients too.

Juice the kale, apple, and pear, and then stir in the spirulina and ground cinnamon at the end.

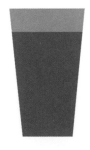

49

GOOD MORNING . . . GOOD DAY

2- to 4-inch piece of fresh ginger
1 cup (250 ml) warm filtered water
juice of 1 lemon
2 tsps ground cinnamon (start off with ½ tsp and work up to this amount)

I tell my clients to start each day with a warm lemon and water drink, and this is my supercharged version. Warming, balancing, and a really lovely way to start out on the right track.

No juicer required. First grate the ginger into a glass, starting small. This is a lot of ginger and may be too strong for a first try! Add the warm water and the lemon juice. Stir in the cinnamon at the end.

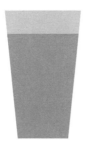

50

FEELING CANDY

**2 handfuls of dandelion
    leaves or spinach**
½ head of broccoli
3 stalks of celery
1 carrot
juice of 1 lemon

High in chromium to help process sugar effectively, this juice is going to provide a huge range of phytonutrients. Dandelion contains inulin, which is helpful in improving blood sugar control. It's a good juice to have as a snack between meals—so put the cookie down, and drink this instead!

If you have hypothyroidism, steam the broccoli before you juice it or replace with extra spinach or Swiss chard.

Pass all the ingredients through the juicer, except the lemon juice, stirring it in at the end.

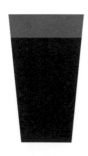

51

I HEART YOU (SMOOTHIE)

¼ cup (25 g) soaked
   and drained oats
15 blueberries
¼ avocado, peeled
   and pitted
2 cups (500 ml)
   coconut water
1–2 tsps chlorella
   powder or spirulina
½ cup (75 g) ice cubes
   (optional)

Oats are an excellent source of fiber, which helps remove unwanted cholesterol from the bowel. The antioxidants in the blueberries and the B vitamins and good fats in the avocado make this a blood pressure– and cholesterol-friendly smoothie. It's a good one for any time and for any reason.

Soak the oats before you make the smoothie for at least 30 minutes or overnight (see page 187). Put all the ingredients into a blender and whiz up.

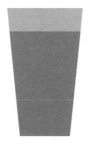

54. Sweet Smiley Sunshine

51. I Heart You

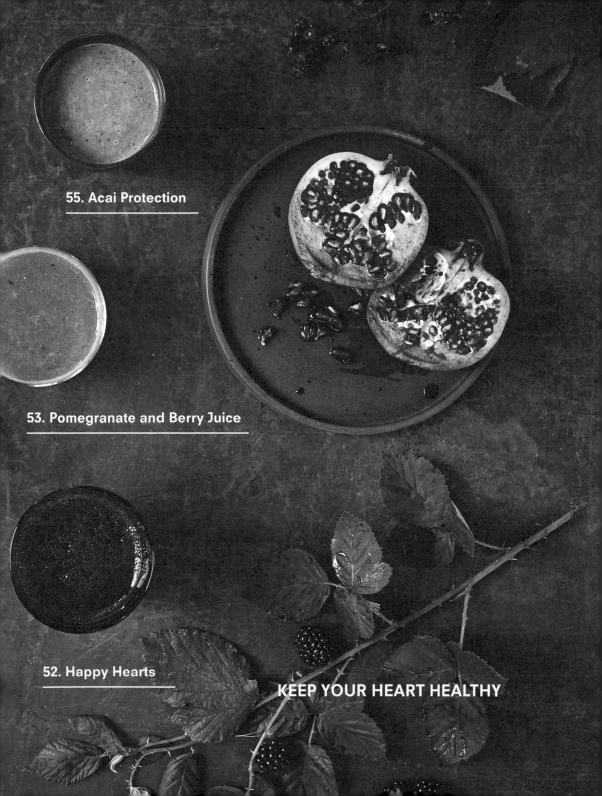

55. Acai Protection

53. Pomegranate and Berry Juice

52. Happy Hearts

KEEP YOUR HEART HEALTHY

52

HAPPY HEARTS

2 carrots
2 stalks of celery
2 beets

A great stabilizing and hydrating juice, this will give you lots of antioxidants. The deep-colored vegetables contain vitamins and minerals that will make your blood pump and your heart sing.

Pass all the ingredients through the juicer.

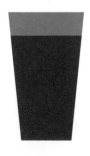

53

POMEGRANATE AND BERRY JUICE

**Seeds from
½ pomegranate
1½ cups (225 g) mixed
    berries
2 apples**

Pomegranate is truly amazing! It is abundant with antioxidants and polyphenols, which are thought to be helpful for the cardiovascular system. So juice away and keep that heart healthy!

Pass all the ingredients through the juicer.

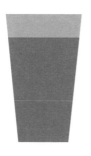

54

SWEET SMILEY SUNSHINE

**½ papaya, peeled
1 passionfruit, peeled
10 blueberries
20 red grapes
juice of 2 oranges**

There is a phytonutrient called hesperidin in oranges, that helps the health of blood vessels, as do the goodies in grapes. Passionfruit is a nutrient powerhouse and gives a lovely sharp kick to juices.

Pass all the ingredients through the juicer, except the orange juice, stirring it in at the end.

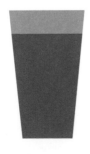

55

ACAI PROTECTION (SMOOTHIE)

½ fennel bulb
1 tbsp chia seeds
2 cups (500 ml)
   unsweetened
   almond milk
2 tsps acai berry
   powder
1 tsp ground turmeric

Acai provides us with the wonderful alpha lipoic acid, which protects by neutralizing free radicals. Almonds are heart friendly too because of the healthy fats they provide, while fennel and turmeric are great for inflammation. We will be helping our bodies to repair with this smoothie.

Put everything into the blender and whiz together.

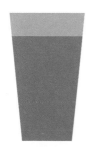

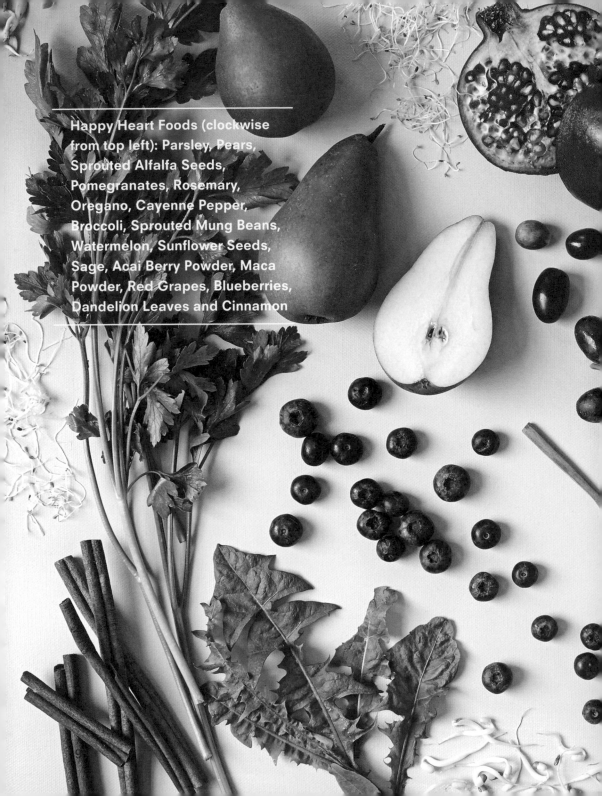

Happy Heart Foods (clockwise from top left): Parsley, Pears, Sprouted Alfalfa Seeds, Pomegranates, Rosemary, Oregano, Cayenne Pepper, Broccoli, Sprouted Mung Beans, Watermelon, Sunflower Seeds, Sage, Acai Berry Powder, Maca Powder, Red Grapes, Blueberries, Dandelion Leaves and Cinnamon

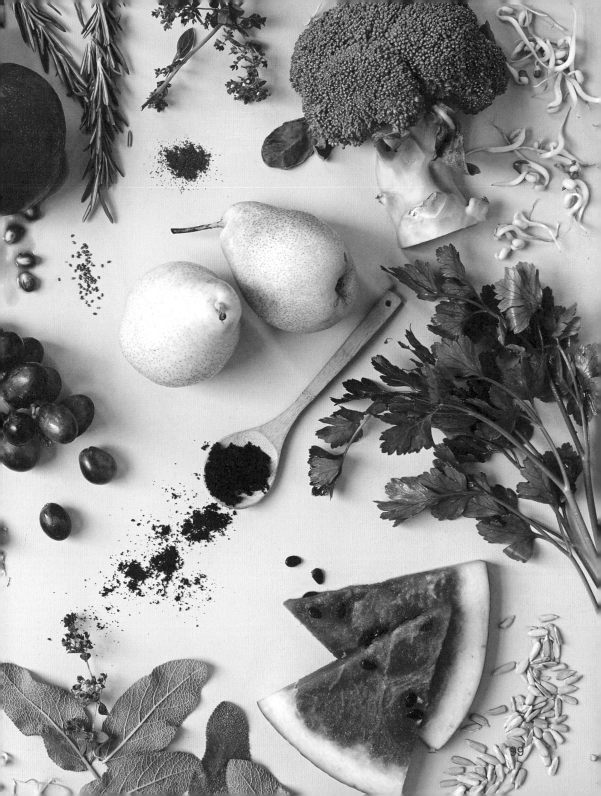

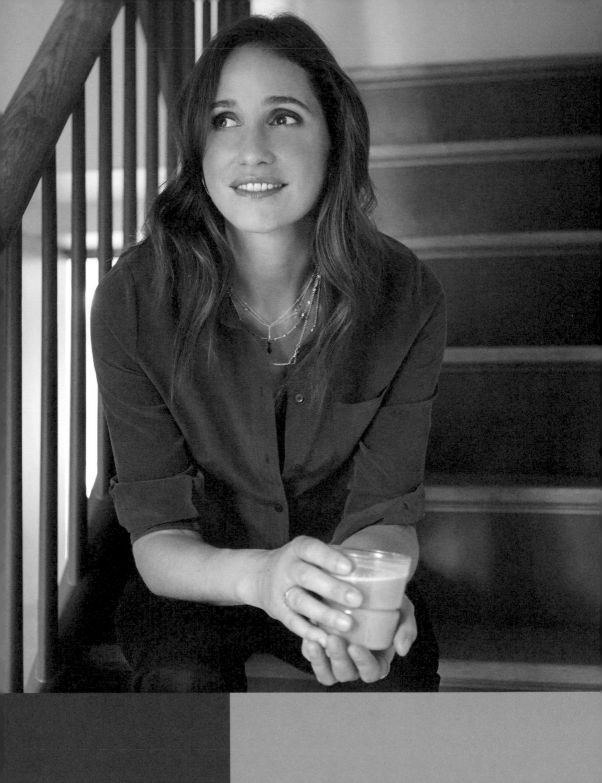

PROTECT
& STRENGTHEN

In this chapter I use ingredients that focus on complementing the body's natural defenses—foods that possess antibacterial and anti-inflammatory properties, foods that are soothing or alkalizing, blood building, and nourishing.

The immune system works tirelessly to protect us from the multitude of viruses and bacteria that threaten to spoil our good health, not to mention protecting us from minor tragedies like spots on the chin or blisters on the feet. A depleted immune system leaves the body vulnerable to acute illnesses like a tummy bug or more serious chronic illnesses that can cause misery for years. Signs of an impaired immunity vary greatly, and can be indicated by repeated illness, inflammation, and general fatigue.

Some of the juices presented in this chapter are specifically designed to help strengthen your immune system, while others are intended to help reduce inflammation and speed up recovery. The job for these juices is to balance the immune system so that it stays fighting fit.

56. Spinach to the Rescue

59. Beet It with Some Garlic

57. Supergree

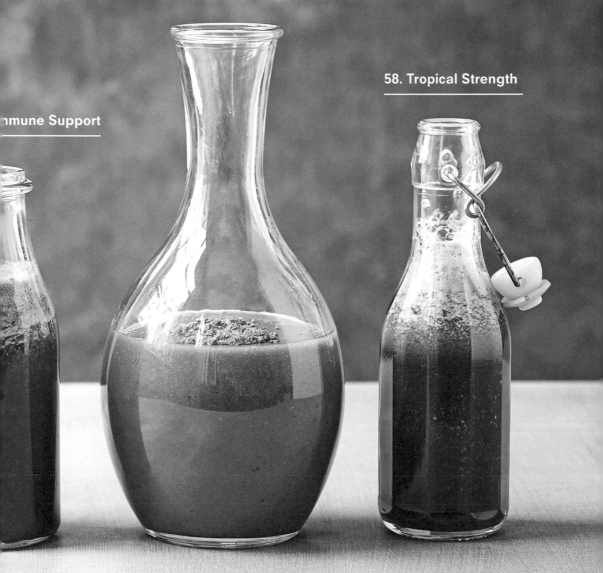

60. Green Iron

58. Tropical Strength

mmune Support

56

SPINACH TO THE RESCUE

1 tsp rosemary leaves
3 large handfuls of
**   spinach**
1 apple
juice of ½ lemon

Simple, straightforward, and effective. Spinach is loaded with nutrients and its vitamin A helps build up white blood cells and fight off any unwanted illnesses. Rosemary is excellent for fighting infection, while lemon alkalizes the body, keeping us in the best possible shape. Apples have the wonderful quercetin, which helps fortify our immune system. As they say, "An apple a day . . . "

Wrap the rosemary in the spinach leaves and pass all the ingredients through the juicer, except the lemon juice, stirring it in at the end.

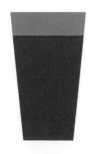

57

SUPERGREEN IMMUNE SUPPORT

4 kale leaves
3 Swiss chard leaves
½ cucumber
2 stalks of celery
handful of parsley
juice of 1–2 limes
1 tsp wheatgrass
   powder

Alkalizing, detoxifying, and blood building, this green juice, while being quite strong, helps support the body's strength by keeping it clean and functioning efficiently. High in chlorophyll and vitamin C, it is an extremely nutrient-dense juice that acts like a protective blanket.

Pass all the ingredients through the juicer, except the lime juice and wheatgrass powder, stirring them in at the end.

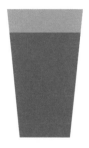

58

TROPICAL STRENGTH (JUICE OR SMOOTHIE)

¼ **watermelon, rind removed**

½ **mango, peeled and pitted**

10 mint leaves

1 tsp matcha green tea powder

This is a lovely refreshing juice. It has a high water content, but you may prefer to blend the ingredients to make a super smoothie—just add ice. The matcha green tea powder certainly makes this an official super juice. It is an amazing powder and fantastic for the immune system. Mango and watermelon not only taste delicious, but are jammed full of phytochemicals that help our bodies stay fit. Happy healthy days!

You can either juice these ingredients, adding the matcha green tea powder at the end, or you can beat them all in a blender and make a smoothie from them!

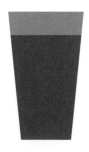

59

BEET IT WITH SOME GARLIC

2 beets
2 apples
1 tsp rosemary leaves
(optional, but
definitely add it
if you are coming
down with a cold—it
is amazing for colds
and the flu)
1 clove of garlic
juice of 2 lemons

This is an immune booster. Garlic is an infection fighter because it is antibacterial, and is particularly helpful for respiratory tract infections. This juice will help stave off any immune invaders and keep those colds at bay.

Pass all the ingredients through the juicer, except the lemon juice, stirring it in at the end. With the garlic, you can either juice it or use a garlic press.

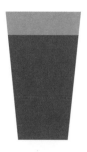

60

GREEN IRON

1 beet
1 apple
1 carrot
¼ head of broccoli
4 lacinato kale leaves
handful of arugula

It makes perfect sense to me that if the body has an abundance of vitamins, minerals, and phytonutrients at its disposal, then it is far more able to cope with the extra pressures it may experience. This juice does just that—it arms you with a serious amount of protection.

If you have hypothyroidism, steam the broccoli before you juice it or replace with spinach or Swiss chard.

Pass all the ingredients through the juicer.

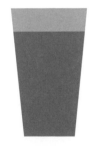

61

A CLASSIC (JUST SQUEEZE, GRATE, AND STIR)

**2-inch piece of fresh
   ginger**
juice of 1 lemon
1 tbsp raw honey
1 tsp ground cinnamon

**To boost this juice you
could add:**
**1 clove of garlic,
   crushed, or/and
   1 tsp rosemary
   leaves**

Comforting and soothing, this juice is for those raw throats and runny noses. The combination of ginger, lemon, honey, and cinnamon work to help clear congestion, to soothe and heal a sore throat, and generally to warm the body. All in all, you'll feel much better for having this. It is a great way to kick-start the day, even if you're not feeling under the weather.

Grate the ginger into a glass and add all the other ingredients, stirring them together.

KEEP COLDS AND COUGHS AT BAY

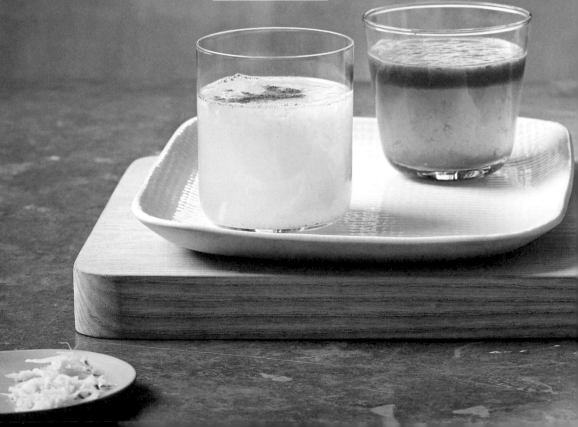

61. A Classic

62. Antiseptic in a Glass

65. Super Herb Helper

64. Virgin Mary

63. Radish Aid

62

ANTISEPTIC IN A GLASS

¼ cabbage
10 oregano leaves
**1- to 2-inch piece of
    fresh ginger**
1 clove of garlic
2 carrots
juice of 2 lemons

When you get that "UH-OH" feeling—the tingle in the nose, the scratch in the throat—this is a go-to juice. Garlic and oregano are nature's antibiotics and will help stave off any incoming illnesses in their early stages. Be brave and add more garlic if you dare . . .

Chop the cabbage into manageable pieces for your juicer. Pass all the ingredients, except the lemon juice, through the juicer, wrapping the oregano in the cabbage leaves. Stir in the lemon juice at the end.

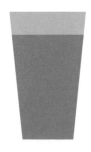

63

RADISH AID

6 radishes
handful of Swiss chard
½ beet
1 red pepper
juice of 2 oranges

Radishes and the other complementary ingredients in this juice are all high in vitamin C, an antioxidant that is super helpful for us when we have a cold. We need to increase our vitamin C when we're sick because when our immune system is killing the infection, free radicals are produced. Vitamin C mops up free radicals and helps us feel better sooner.

Pass all the ingredients through the juicer, except the orange juice, stirring it in at the end.

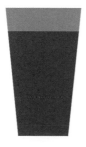

64

VIRGIN MARY

4 tomatoes
2 stalks of celery
1 apple
2-inch piece of fresh
    horseradish or
    2 tsps prepared
    horseradish
juice of 1 lemon
1 tsp Himalayan crystal
    salt

Sounds familiar? Perhaps with vodka! But maybe you haven't realized the benefits of a Virgin Mary made with fresh ingredients. Horseradish helps to get rid of unwanted bacteria, and aids digestion too. The crystal salt helps hydration levels if we're suffering with a fever, as it acts as an electrolyte and also provides minerals. This juice also has good amounts of vitamins and phytonutrients, all of which will help you to recover faster!

Pass all the ingredients, except the lemon juice and salt, through the juicer. Stir in the lemon juice and salt at the end.

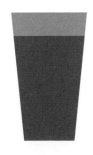

65

SUPER HERB HELPER (JUICE OR SMOOTHIE)

handful of mint leaves
1 zucchini
1 apple
1- to 2-inch piece of
**   fresh ginger**
juice of 1 lemon
1 tsp matcha green
**   tea powder**
1 tsp ground turmeric
1 tsp ground cardamom
1 tsp raw honey
pinch of Himalayan
**   crystal salt**

If you are feeling congested mentally or physically, this should help to clear it! The juice uses powerful herbs to help stimulate your system, clears the airways, and relieves any tension in the body.

Juice the mint, zucchini, apple, and ginger, and stir in the lemon juice. Add the matcha green tea powder, turmeric, cardamom, honey, and crystal salt at the end, or you can whiz it all in the blender and make a smoothie.

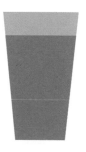

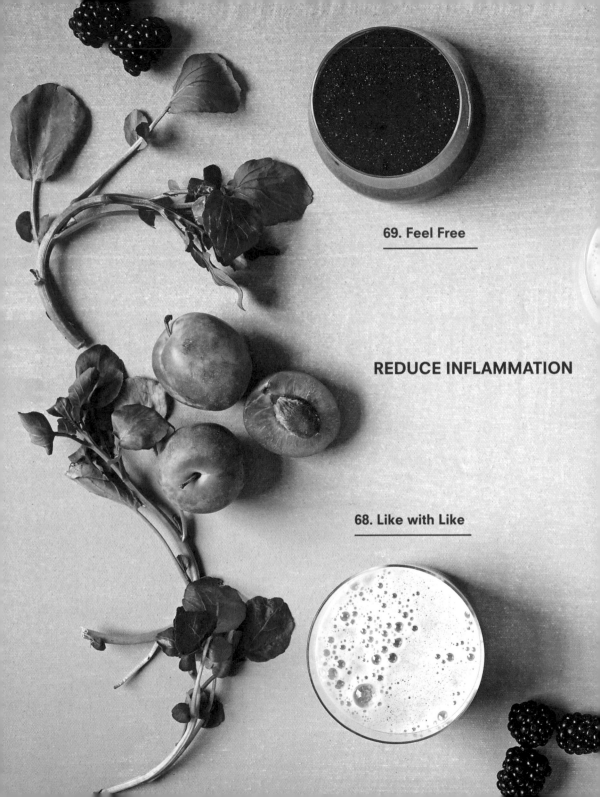

69. Feel Free

REDUCE INFLAMMATION

68. Like with Like

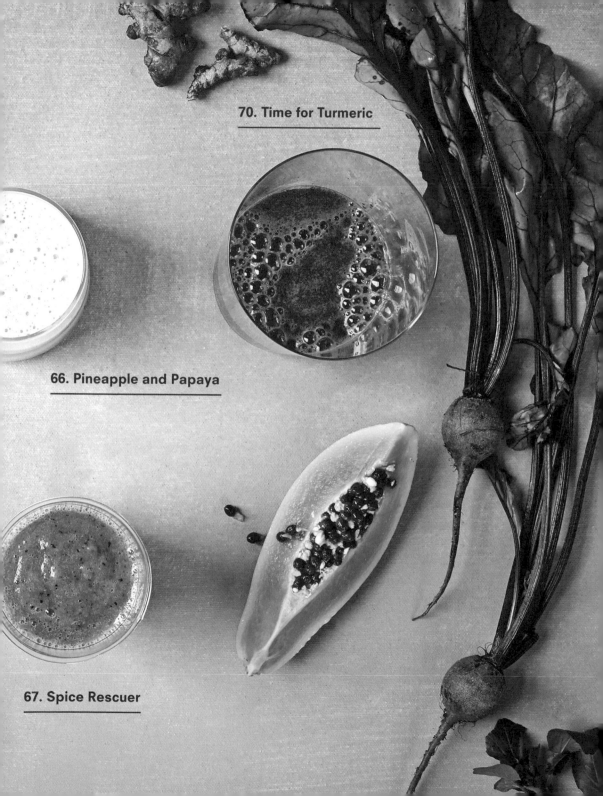

70. Time for Turmeric

66. Pineapple and Papaya

67. Spice Rescuer

66

PINEAPPLE AND PAPAYA

½ **papaya, peeled**
¼ **pineapple, rind**
    removed
2 stalks of celery
handful of parsley

Pineapple contains bromelain, which can have positive anti-inflammatory effects. Add the papaya, celery, and parsley and you have a juice that is alkalizing and full of soluble fiber. An acidic body can cause inflammation in joints and tissues. This juice will address this and help to relieve any inflammation we might have.

Pass all the ingredients through the juicer.

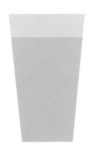

67

SPICE RESCUER (SMOOTHIE)

¼ **papaya, peeled**
10 blueberries
small handful of
    spinach
1- to 2-inch piece of
    fresh ginger
½ **tsp ground turmeric**
¼ **tsp cayenne pepper**
¼ **tsp ground cinnamon**
1 tbsp flaxseed oil
1 cup (250 ml)
    coconut water

Turmeric, cayenne, cinnamon, papaya, ginger, flaxseed oil, and coconut make up an all-star anti-inflammatory cast. Omega 3 in the flaxseed oil, gives the body a greater chance of following an anti-inflammatory pathway. The heat from the spices actually calms any hotspots in the body, whether on the skin, in the joints, or wherever there is inflammation.

Put all the ingredients into the blender and give them a good whiz!

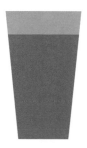

68

LIKE WITH LIKE

¼ **cabbage, chopped into manageable pieces for your juicer**
small handful of watercress
small handful of parsley
2 stalks of celery
2 apples
2- to 4-inch piece of fresh ginger (add more if you can!)

The more ginger you can handle, the better it is! "Like with Like" is a powerful anti-inflammatory juice and can also provide some pain relief. I love the way it tastes, but it can get quite hot, so build it up gently. By juicing green vegetables, you're ingesting more volume than you could by eating them. The vegetables will re-alkalize your system, while the antioxidant apples contain quercetin, which can help reduce inflammation.

Pass all the ingredients through the juicer and enjoy!

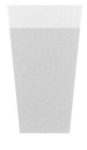

69

FEEL FREE (SMOOTHIE)

4 plums, pitted
6 cherries, pitted
8 blackberries
1 tbsp chia seeds
1 tbsp aloe vera juice
1–2 cups (250–500 ml) unsweetened almond milk
2 tbsps mixed green powder (a mix of spirulina, chlorella, wheatgrass, etc.)

Plums and blackberries can help mobilize uric acid away from the joints, therefore helping with stiffness or gout-like symptoms. Loaded with omega 3 and other alkalizing ingredients, this juice should help get inflammation under control, and get you on the road to feeling amazing!

Put all other ingredients, except the green powder, in the blender and whiz up. Stir in the green powder at the end.

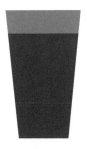

70

TIME FOR TURMERIC

1 apple
1 pear
1 carrot
½ beet
small handful of
   cilantro
2-inch piece of fresh
   ginger
2- to 4-inch piece of
   fresh turmeric
   or 1–2 tsps
   ground turmeric
juice of 1–2 lemons

This is a lovely all-around juice, with great anti-inflammatory power. Turmeric is such an amazing spice—while fresh is better, it's not always easy to find. Use whatever form is available to you and add more than the recommended amounts if you want to.

Juice all the ingredients together, except the lemon juice, stirring it in at the end. If you have fresh turmeric, then juice that too. If not, then stir in the powder at the end.

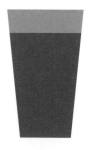

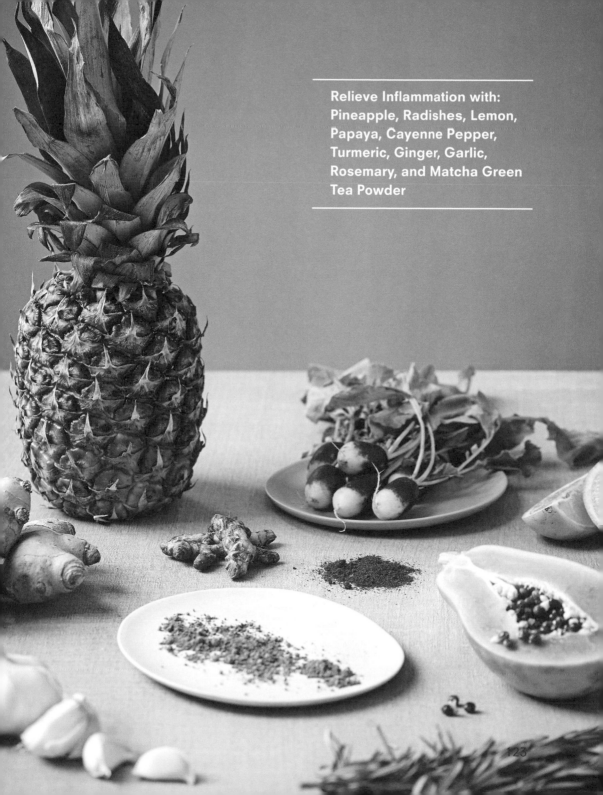

**Relieve Inflammation with:
Pineapple, Radishes, Lemon,
Papaya, Cayenne Pepper,
Turmeric, Ginger, Garlic,
Rosemary, and Matcha Green
Tea Powder**

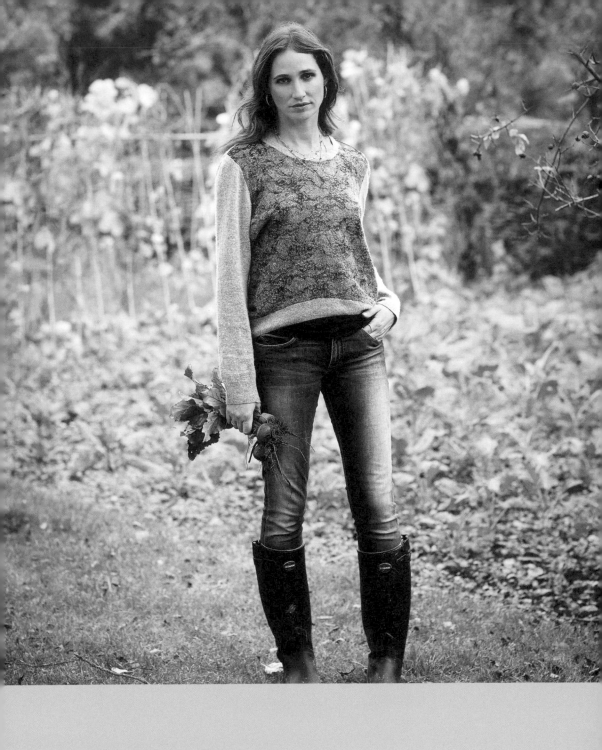

CALM
& BALANCE

Hormones are chemical messengers in the body. They are produced by endocrine glands such as the adrenals and reproductive organs. Stress, among many other things, can deplete these glands of the nutrition they need to function correctly, so this group of juices contains nutrients that support a healthy hormone balance for men and women.

The thyroid is crucial for the regulation of the metabolic rate, and if it is low a person can feel sluggish, tired, and irritable and suffer noticeable hair loss.

Many people suffer with other hormonal problems, such as premenstrual syndrome (PMS), prostate problems, and menopause. This chapter is aimed at supporting the hormone balances in the body that keep us feeling energetic and balanced.

71. Apple and Chard

72. B6 Power

75. Juice for Change

77. Thyroid-Friendly Green

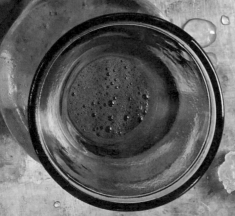

76. Thyroid Helper

74. Jolly Juice

BALANCING FEMALE HORMONES

73. Wonderful Juice

71

APPLE AND CHARD

2 apples
3 Swiss chard leaves
¼ fennel bulb
handful of parsley
juice of 1 lemon

Phytoestrogens are found in these ingredients and many other plants too. They are useful when we are experiencing PMS. During menopause, these ingredients can also reduce symptoms of lowered estrogen. The green leafy vegetables in this juice also provide a vitamin B6 boost and help the liver remove unwanted hormones from the body.

Pass all the ingredients through the juicer, except the lemon juice, stirring it in at the end.

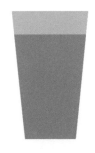

72

B6 POWER (SMOOTHIE)

½ **avocado, peeled and pitted**
½ **banana, peeled**
1 tbsp sunflower seeds
5 walnuts
½ **carrot**
1 cup (250 ml) unsweetened almond or oat milk
1 cup (250 ml) filtered water or
  1 cup (150 g) ice cubes

Vitamin B6 is a very supportive vitamin for PMS. It can help with water retention, support oxygen flow, and support optimal hormone levels. B vitamins, especially B6, can also help if you suffer with tenderness and cramps. This smoothie is high in essential fatty acids, which help to regulate female reproductive organs. So if you're feeling weak or uncomfortable, try this. It's a lovely, nourishing smoothie, and pretty comforting too.

Put all the ingredients into the blender and whiz them together.

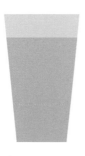

73

WONDERFUL JUICE

6 dandelion leaves
handful of spinach
2 carrots
1 red pepper
1 tsp sesame seeds

This juice is full of nutrients that support the liver and the removal of excess hormones from the body. The dandelion leaves have a diuretic action, so they help if water retention is a problem, as well as being supportive to blood sugar balance, so hopefully this juice will ease those sugar cravings around the time of the month. On top of all that, we have sesame, which gives us calcium and is really important, ladies, because of osteoporosis.

Pass all the ingredients, except the sesame seeds, through a juicer, and then stir in the sesame seeds at the end.

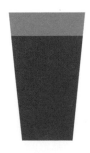

74

JOLLY JUICE

½ **pineapple, rind removed**
½ **cucumber**
handful of spinach
½ **fennel bulb**
juice of 1 lime

This juice can help if you suffer from cramping or bloating. Spinach is packed with magnesium, which is a natural relaxer and soothing to the tummy. Fennel helps to relieve bloating, and also control those dreaded sugar cravings. This is a good "mood food" juice, especially at a time of the month when you may be feeling less than jolly.

Pass all ingredients through the juicer, except the lime juice, stirring it in at the end.

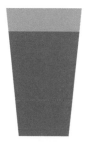

75

JUICE FOR CHANGE

10 raspberries
1 beet
handful of spinach
small handful of
    watercress
6 sage leaves
juice of 1 lemon

An excellent juice to counteract those hot flashes. I've had great clinical results with sage managing menopausal symptoms. It is such an easy herb to buy or grow. This juice also has a bit of calcium and magnesium, some antioxidants, and some phytoestrogens . . . and . . . and . . . and! It's really good—even if you're not menopausal (or you're male).

Pass all the ingredients through the juicer, except the lemon juice, stirring it in at the end.

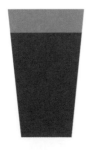

76

THYROID HELPER

¼ **watermelon, rind removed**
½ **globe artichoke, stalk and outer leaves removed**
½ **leek**
1 **red pepper**
1 **tbsp aloe vera juice**

This may sound like an odd juice, but the ingredients have been selected for good reason. Iodine is essential for the thyroid to work properly, and leeks and artichokes are rich in iodine. You can always add a pinch of iodized salt to your juice, too. Aloe is generally very soothing, brings balance to the body, and helps cleanse and heal the system.

Pass the watermelon and artichoke along with the leek and red pepper through the juicer, then stir in the aloe vera juice at the end.

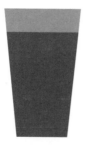

77

THYROID-FRIENDLY GREEN (SMOOTHIE)

**½ avocado, peeled and
    pitted**
1 stalk of celery
½ apple
juice of ½ lemon
1 tbsp pumpkin seeds
**2 cups (500 ml)
    coconut water**

Packed with essential fatty acids and thyroid-friendly nutrients such as L-tyrosine, selenium, and zinc, this smoothie will help balance the thyroid and give it the nutrition it needs to work optimally—hopefully making you feel full of life.

Add all the ingredients to the blender and whiz together.

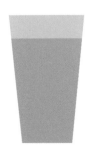

78

PROTECT AND STRENGTHEN

¼ **watermelon, rind removed**
½ **grapefruit, peeled**
4 Swiss chard leaves
handful of arugula

Both watermelon and grapefruit have high levels of the antioxidant lycopene. The dark leafy greens—the chard and arugula—are full of B vitamins, making this juice supportive to the prostate and male hormone levels.

Pass all the ingredients through the juicer.

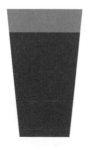

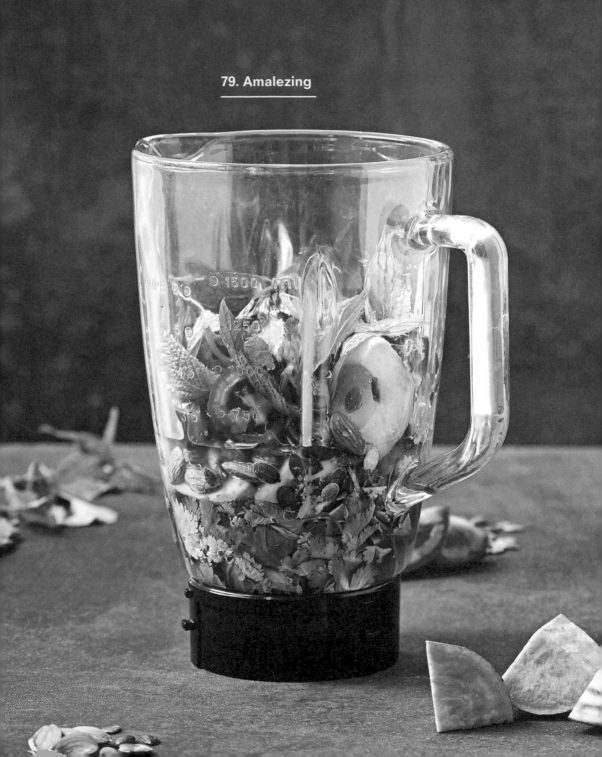

BALANCING MALE HORMONES

80. Well Man Juice

78. Protect and Strengthen

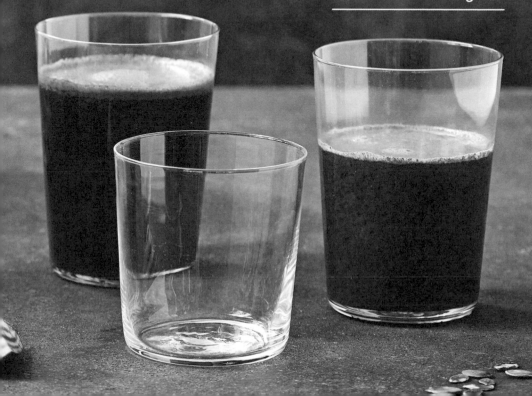

79

AMALEZING (SMOOTHIE)

**1 small avocado,
   peeled and pitted**
½ banana, peeled
2 tomatoes
5 almonds
1 tsp pumpkin seeds
**small handful of
   cilantro**
juice of 1 lime
**small handful of mint
   leaves**
**1 cup (250 ml)
   coconut water**

This sounds like a recipe for a sort of guacamole. And I'm sure it would make great dip, but we are going to whiz it up with some coconut water to make a wonderful male hormone-supporting smoothie instead. The avocado, almonds, and pumpkin seeds are packed with beta-sitosterol, which is a plant-derived fat that has been shown to help symptoms associated with an enlarged prostate. Pumpkin seeds are high in zinc, which is essential for all matters related to the prostate, and the tomatoes bring lycopene, a very protective antioxidant for the men among us.

Put all the ingredients into the blender and whiz together.

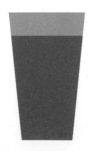

80

WELL MAN JUICE

¼ **head of broccoli**
handful of spinach
1 beet
1 sweet potato
10 red grapes
2- to 4-inch piece of fresh ginger (this is a lot of ginger, so start small and see how you do)

This combination of ingredients makes an anti-inflammatory, high in B vitamin, zinc-providing juice. It's not only protective behind the scenes, but will also leave you feeling energized and cared for!

If you have hypothyroidism, steam the broccoli before you juice it or replace with extra spinach or Swiss chard.

Pass all the ingredients through the juicer.

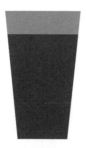

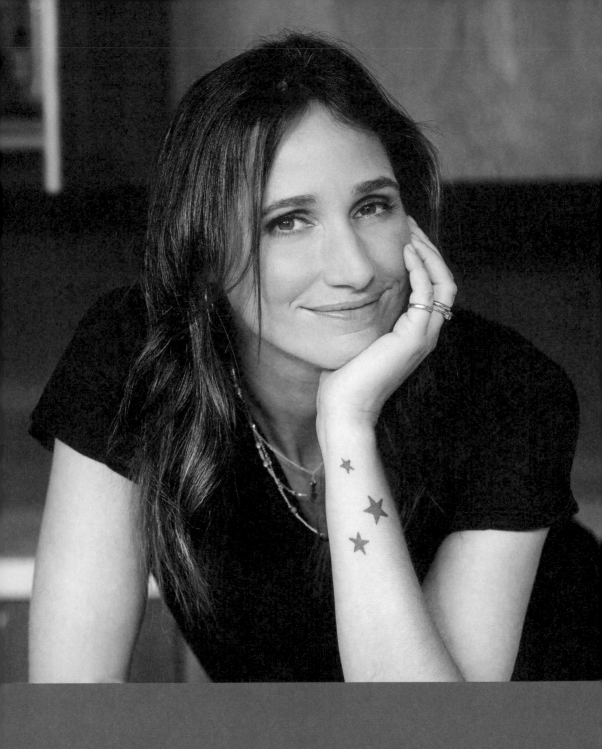

CARE
& PRESERVE

Being beautiful inside and out should be a natural given, but would your body agree? I hope this section of the book demonstrates that you need to protect the inside if you want to look good on the outside, not simply for cosmetic reasons, but because feeling vibrant shines from the inside out and gives you your natural glow.

Being overweight can create a host of problems, physical and psychological, while pushing yourself at the gym without the proper nutrient profile will leave you feeling rough and in pain. In this chapter there are juices and smoothies that will help you to stay fuller for longer, and therefore reduce your urge to reach for high-fat or sugary processed foods. The "workout" recipes will give you nutrients that work with your body as you get fitter, helping to repair the body after a workout and mop up the free radicals that doing exercise can create.

Dry or problem skin is never simply skin-deep, but usually an indication that something else is going on. By encouraging the elimination of waste, making sure you drink enough water, and taking in higher levels of antioxidants, essential fatty acids, and phytonutrients, your skin will benefit and you will feel lighter and more energized.

Juicing is a step in the right direction toward feeling beautiful inside and out. By giving yourself a chance to feel more positive, you will more likely be motivated to do that 10K run or lose weight, rather than remaining lethargic because of unhealthy foods that negatively impact your body's system.

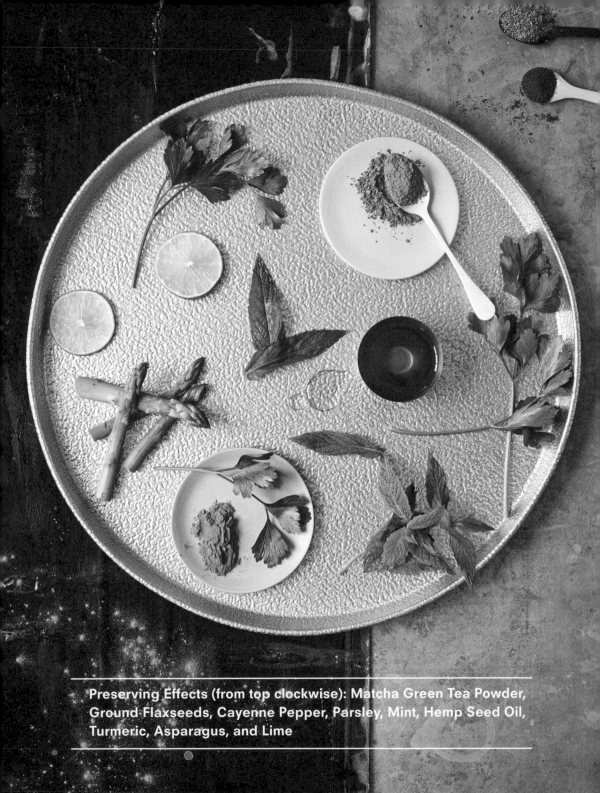

Preserving Effects (from top clockwise): Matcha Green Tea Powder, Ground Flaxseeds, Cayenne Pepper, Parsley, Mint, Hemp Seed Oil, Turmeric, Asparagus, and Lime

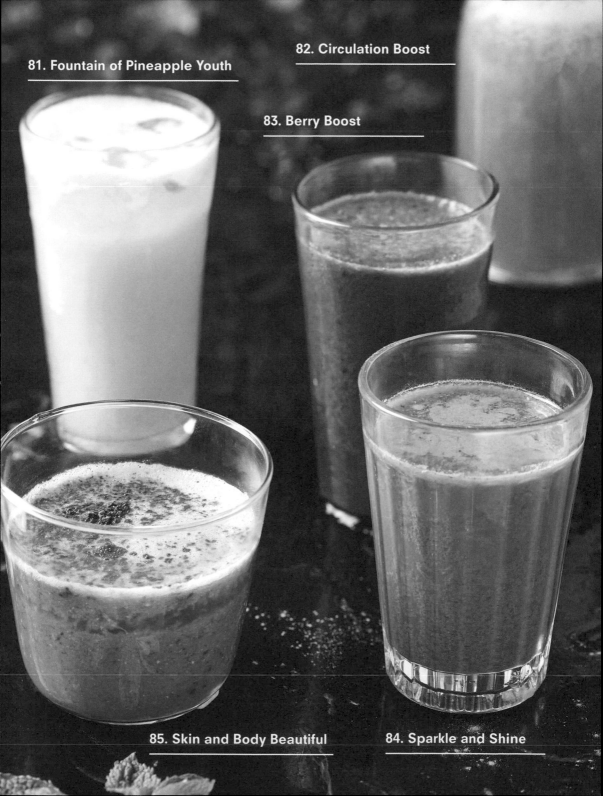

81. Fountain of Pineapple Youth

82. Circulation Boost

83. Berry Boost

85. Skin and Body Beautiful

84. Sparkle and Shine

81

FOUNTAIN OF PINEAPPLE YOUTH

**1 pineapple, peeled
juice of 1 orange
2 tbsps hemp seed oil**

This juice is full of minerals and also contains essential fatty acids, which help skin retain its tone and brightness. The pineapple's anti-inflammatory properties will also help keep skin smooth, while the vitamin C in this juice will plump up the natural collagen, keeping you looking youthful at a cellular level.

Juice the pineapple, then stir in the orange juice and hemp seed oil at the end.

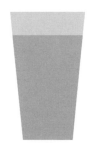

82

CIRCULATION BOOST

½ **honeydew melon,**
   rind removed
1 pear
1 apple
handful of mint
1 tsp cayenne pepper
   (work up to this
   amount, start small!)

Honeydew melon has a good amount of copper and works with the vitamin C contained in this juice to aid the production of collagen. The cayenne and mint are amazing for circulation, boosting blood flow to the skin and helping to clear any problem areas.

Pass all ingredients through the juicer, except the cayenne pepper, stirring it in at the end.

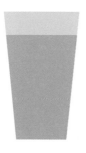

83

BERRY BOOST

10 raspberries
10 blueberries
5 strawberries
1 carrot
handful of parsley
¼ fennel bulb

Bursting with antioxidants, this will help rid the body of toxins that make you look tired. If you're looking tired, then you're probably feeling tired, so give yourself a boost! This juice is a ray of sunshine in a glass.

Pass all the ingredients through the juicer.

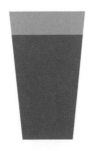

84

SPARKLE AND SHINE

2 apricots, pitted
10 raspberries
2 carrots
handful of spring
    greens
1 tsp ground turmeric

Lovely and sweet, with the earthy taste of turmeric. This juice will protect the cells from free radical damage. It is an eye-bright recipe too, with the carrots and apricots helping the eyes to sparkle!

Pass all the ingredients, except the turmeric, through the juicer. Stir in the turmeric at the end and work up to the recommended amount—you may find the taste quite strong at first.

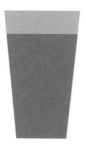

85

SKIN AND BODY BEAUTIFUL

¼ **head of broccoli**
½ **head of romaine**
 lettuce
2 spears of asparagus
handful of spinach
1 stalk of celery
juice of 1 lime
juice of 1 orange
2 tsps matcha green
 tea powder

This is a strong-tasting juice—be warned! Hydrating and high in silica, with folic acid and vitamin E, this is a blood-building juice that protects the skin from the inside out. It helps the skin to remain supple and fresh while delivering the nutrients we need. Matcha green tea powder is packed with antioxidants and other compounds, which are fabulously helpful to counter signs of aging in both skin and body.

If you have hypothyroidism, steam the broccoli before you juice it or replace with spinach or Swiss chard.

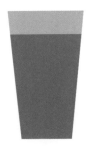

Pass all the ingredients through the juicer, except the lime and orange juice and matcha green tea powder, stirring them in at the end.

86

PRE-SUN JUICE

1 papaya, peeled
2 tomatoes
2 carrots
juice of 1 orange
juice of 1 lime
1 tsp cayenne pepper
   (optional if you
   prefer a bit less
   heat)

Tomatoes and papaya are high in lycopene and beta-carotene, a form of vitamin A. These little nutrients are big on protecting your skin from long spells in the sun. Of course you still need that SPF 30 sunscreen, but your skin should be in better shape than it would without this juice!

Pass all the ingredients through the juicer, except the lime and orange juice and cayenne pepper, stirring them in at the end.

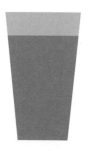

HEALTHY INSIDE, HEALTHY ON THE OUTSIDE

90. Simple Skin Saver

86. Pre-sun Juice

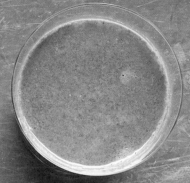

89. Clean and Strengthen

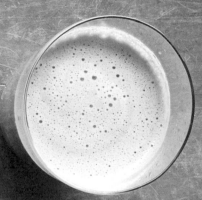

87. Skin Healer

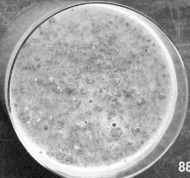

88. Hydration Station

87

SKIN HEALER (SMOOTHIE)

3 plums, pitted
1 tbsp flaxseed or
  evening primrose oil
small handful of Swiss
  chard
2 dandelion leaves
5 strawberries
2 tsps pumpkin seeds
½ cup (125 ml)
  unsweetened
  almond milk
½ cup (75 g) ice cubes

Your skin will be glowing with this smoothie. It has some zinc to heal any breakouts, and its essential fatty acids are perfect for smooth, soft skin and tissue repair. Plums and strawberries pump up the antioxidants; clean on the inside, shows on the outside!

Place all the ingredients into your blender and whiz up.

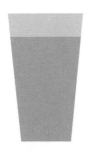

88

HYDRATION STATION

¼ **tbsp soaked and drained chia seeds (to supercharge the hydrating quality of this juice)**
1 **peach, pitted**
½ **cucumber**
2 **stalks of celery**
1 **carrot**
2 **apples**

The ingredients in this juice are full of water and the minerals that help the body absorb moisture. It's a simple, quick route to hydrating your skin from the inside.

Soak the chia seeds before you make the smoothie for at least 30 minutes or overnight (see page 187). Pass all the ingredients, except the chia seeds, through the juicer. Stir in the soaked chia seeds after you have made the juice.

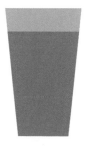

89

CLEAN AND STRENGTHEN

**small handful of
   cilantro
handful of kale
handful of watercress
2 carrots
juice of 2 oranges**

Great for skin and hair, the B vitamins in the greens help detoxify the body and leave the way clear to build healthy glossy hair. Beautiful skin is boosted by the oranges, which are high in vitamin C—essential for collagen repair.
The vitamin A in the carrots helps strengthen the skin tissue.

Pass all the ingredients through the juicer, except the orange juice, stirring it in at the end.

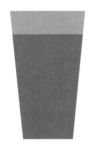

90

SIMPLE SKIN SAVER

1 apple
1 carrot
20 blueberries
handful of parsley
2- to 4-inch piece of
fresh ginger

Simply a fantastic all-around skin juice. It is anti-aging and has soluble fiber to help the body's elimination of toxins. It's hydrating, full of antioxidants, and the ginger will help the circulation and therefore help the blood remove toxins that lurk under the skin.

Pass all the ingredients through the juicer.

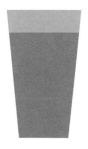

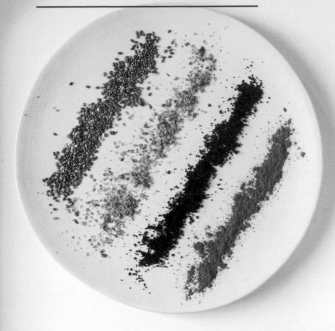

Left to Right: Chia Seeds, Ground Flaxseeds, Acai Berry Powder, and Cinnamon

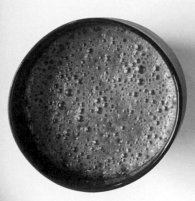

91. Feeling Light

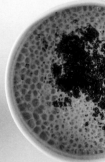

95. Fuller for Longer

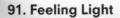

HELPFUL AIDS FOR
WEIGHT MANAGEMENT

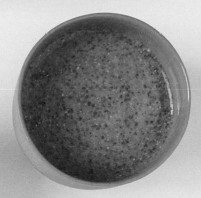

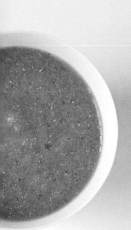

93. On the Right Track

92. Fiber Fullness

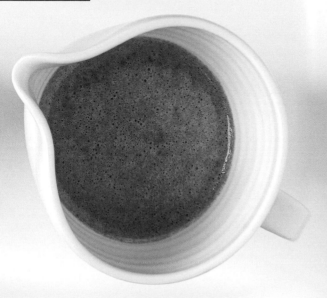

94. Spice It Up

91

FEELING LIGHT

¼ pineapple, rind removed
½ cucumber
2 stalks of celery
2 tsps acai berry powder

This is the most delicious juice! It is uplifting, hydrating, and detoxing—all the things required to drop a few pounds. Acai is well known for helping with weight management because it gives the metabolism a real boost. If you're feeling positive, you're far more likely to take care of yourself. Eating fresh fruit and veg will let you detox and lose weight simultaneously.

Juice all the ingredients, except the acai berry powder, adding it at the end.

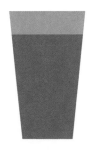

92

FIBER FULLNESS (SMOOTHIE)

⅓ **banana, peeled**
small handful of
**   spinach**
3 spears of asparagus
1 tbsp flaxseeds
1 tsp ground cinnamon
2 cups (500 ml)
**   filtered water**

Fiber is essential for the body to remove waste products easily and it also assists with the removal of toxins. In turn, we will release any water we're retaining as well as begin to shed excess weight. Because this smoothie is high in fiber, we should feel fuller for longer, keeping our blood sugar and energy on a level.

Blend all the ingredients together.

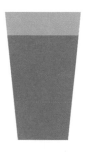

93

ON THE RIGHT TRACK

1 nectarine, pitted
2 kiwifruits
1 apple
¼ pineapple, rind removed

Although this is purely a fruit juice, it has some serious ingredients to help the body let go of surplus weight. The soluble fiber pectin, found in apples, is great because the fiber encourages waste removal from the body. The low glycemic index of kiwi, and the antioxidant power in all the individual elements, make this an ideal alternative to sugary, processed snacks. It's a real pick-me-up and will keep you on the straight and narrow.

Peel the kiwifruit if you prefer, then juice all the ingredients together.

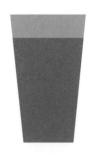

94

SPICE IT UP

2 carrots
½ cucumber
1 apple
½ fresh chile pepper, deseeded (you may want to start with less, it can get quite spicy!)

This juice is thermogenic, which means that it creates heat in the body and it will nudge up your metabolism. You can turn up the heat in this juice by adding more fresh chile.

Juice all the ingredients together.

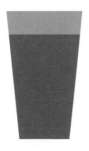

95

FULLER FOR LONGER (SMOOTHIE)

½ avocado, peeled and
    pitted
½ grapefruit, peeled
10 blueberries
1 tbsp chia seeds
1 cup (250 ml) filtered
    water

This smoothie will keep you feeling fuller for longer. Avocado contains oleic acid, a monounsaturated fat that, along with the protein content, may actually slow your hunger. Grapefruit contains a flavonoid called naringin, which is good for levels of red blood cells. High in fiber and hydration, this smoothie will keep you going for a while, and would be good as a substantial snack.

Blend all the ingredients together.

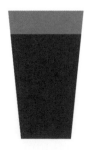

96

PRE-CLASS (SMOOTHIE)

½ **avocado, peeled and pitted**
½ **peach, pitted**
1½ **cups (375 ml) unsweetened almond milk**
handful of parsley
juice of 1 orange
1 **tsp wheatgrass powder**
1 **tsp maca powder**

This smoothie will help your energy levels during exercise class and also delivers the enzyme carnitine to you via the avocado. It helps you burn fat and feel energetic throughout a tough training session. Remember to leave time for your smoothie to digest before your workout. It needs to be digested so that the nutrients have been broken down and are ready to get to work, not sloshing around in your stomach!

Place all the ingredients into the blender and whiz them up.

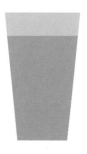

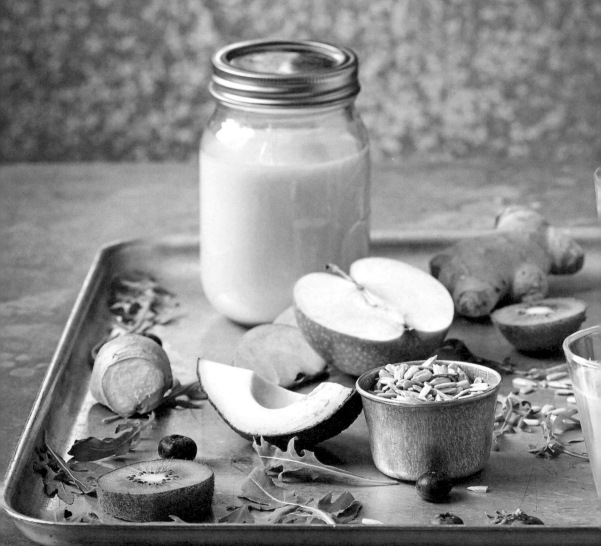

97. Feel the Burn

96. Pre-class

100. Reenergize and Repair

99. Rainbow Juice

98. Nutrient Power

97

FEEL THE BURN

½ cucumber
3 stalks of celery
   handful of Swiss
   chard
1 apple
2-inch piece of fresh
   ginger
juice of ½ lemon
1 tsp cayenne pepper
   (or to your taste)

After you have sweated it out in the gym, this juice is great for rehydration because of the celery and cucumber. The silica in cucumber is great for joint health, and, best of all, the cayenne pepper will keep your metabolism going at a faster pace once you leave the gym, so you'll actually continue burning calories!

Pass all the ingredients through the juicer, except the lemon juice and cayenne pepper, stirring them in at the end. Start small when adding the cayenne—you don't want it to be too overwhelming.

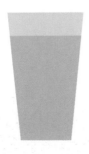

98

NUTRIENT POWER (SMOOTHIE)

1 banana, peeled
10 blueberries
5 strawberries
1 tsp sunflower seeds
1 tsp flaxseeds
1 tsp chlorella powder
   or spirulina
1½ cups (375 ml)
   unsweetened
   almond milk or
   filtered water
1 tsp maca powder

This is an amazing muscle repair and revive smoothie, high in protein, fiber, B vitamins, and slow-burning energy. It replaces many of the nutrients used up while exercising, so you should feel totally nourished by this.

Put all the ingredients into the blender and whiz them up. All done!

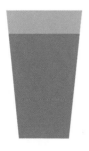

99

RAINBOW JUICE

½ beet
1 carrot
handful of spinach
5 strawberries
10 blueberries
juice of ½ lemon
2 tsps blue green algae

This is a multivitamin in a glass! It contains all the colors of the rainbow, so you are getting a whole spectrum of antioxidants, vitamins, and minerals— all necessary to heal and repair the body. The live enzymes in the blue green algae, plus the B12, will leave you feeling totally regenerated after your yoga class!

Pass all the ingredients through the juicer, except the lemon juice and blue green algae, stirring them in at the end.

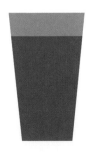

100

REENERGIZE AND REPAIR

1 kiwifruit
½ head of broccoli
1 pear
1 apple
handful of arugula

This is a real little energy boost for you before or after you've worked out. It will help repair any damage, and the greens will support the liver to neutralize any free radicals created by your hard workout.

If you have hypothyroidism, steam the broccoli before you juice it or replace with spinach or Swiss chard.

It is up to you whether you prefer to peel your kiwifruit or not, you can juice it either way. Pass all the ingredients through the juicer.

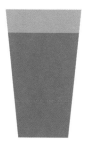

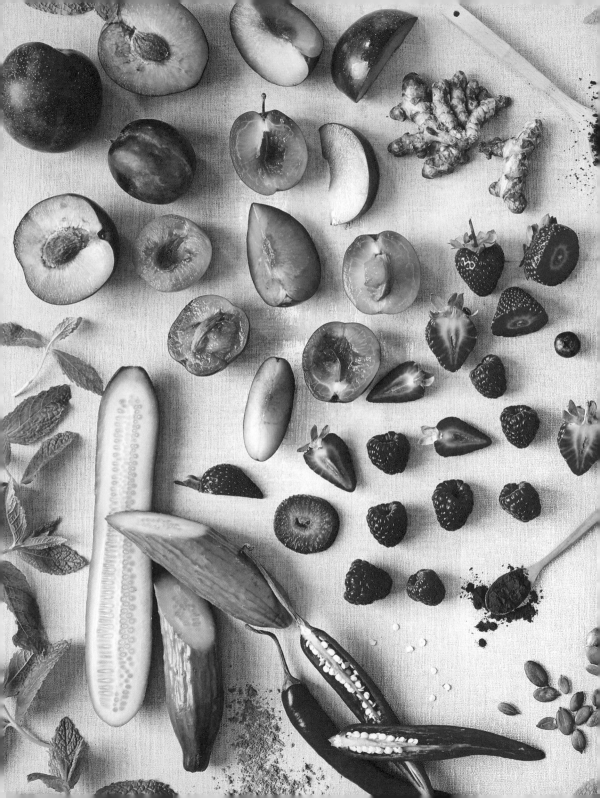

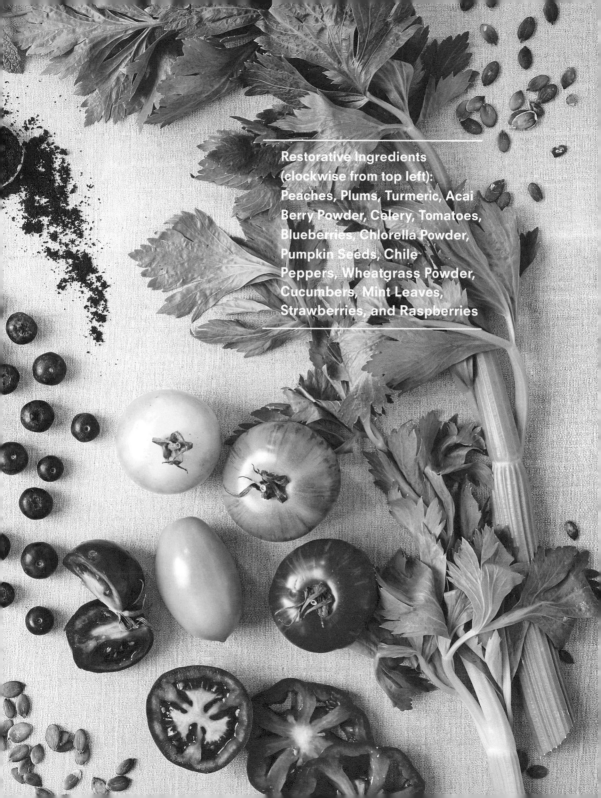

Restorative Ingredients
(clockwise from top left):
Peaches, Plums, Turmeric, Acai
Berry Powder, Celery, Tomatoes,
Blueberries, Chlorella Powder,
Pumpkin Seeds, Chile
Peppers, Wheatgrass Powder,
Cucumbers, Mint Leaves,
Strawberries, and Raspberries

MY DETOX PLANS

JUICE FASTING

Fasting may be one of the oldest forms of healthcare there is! When sickness hits us, many of us do not feel like eating at all. We rest and conserve our energy to heal the body. Eating, chewing, and digesting food takes 50 percent of our energy every day, so it makes sense to me that by not taking in food for a day or 3, we will have 50 percent more energy to heal and repair other areas of our body.

We are going to focus on detoxing through liquid fasting. By using juices and smoothies that encourage the toxins out of the tissue and into the bloodstream, we can then excrete them from our body and achieve a lower toxic load. There are many benefits to detoxing, including higher energy, weight loss, alertness, mental sharpness, better sleep, anti-aging, better transit time, and water retention among many others.

I try to fast 1 day every week. If you can do this too, by the end of the year you will have done 52 days of fasting. Obviously this doesn't happen every week for me, life isn't that straightforward, but I do try. For me personally, it helps me to stay on the "straight and narrow," reminding me to eat clean food, especially if I have had a less than ideal weekend! Yes, I do this on a Monday to start the week with a bang. It really sets me on the right track and gets my energy and positivity levels up.

For a more intense cleanse, juice fasting for 2 or 3 days goes deeper. It is more committed and needs more willpower. I tend to do longer fasts after holiday seasons when I haven't been able, or wanted, to do a weekly fast. A 2-day fast is great if you can't do a weekly detox. It is more concentrated and you could do this once a month. The 3-day plan is a twice-a-year event. It may be tough, but you do feel very rejuvenated afterward. It will allow your gut and bowel to have a complete rest, and encourage cleansing of the colon. It is not only your body that starts to feel lighter, clearer, and more energized; your mind can become very clear too.

THINGS TO BE AWARE OF

Pick the right day or days to detox. There is no point doing it if you are meeting friends for dinner, or have the busiest day of the year. That being said, you absolutely can do the 1- and 2-day detoxes when you are at work.

You will be fine to go to the gym too; just try doing a more restorative form of exercise such as yoga. Moving the body gets the lymph moving and encourages toxins to leave the tissue so they can be expelled from the body.

It is not good to do a detox with a hangover because the amount of toxins in your system could make you feel very unwell, as they will leave the body at a faster rate.

Detoxing can cause feelings of nausea, headaches, body odor, skin rashes, a coated tongue, a change in bowel movements, and fatigue. Any symptoms of detoxing are just a sign of the toxins leaving the tissue, hitting the bloodstream and making you feel yucky. Obviously you should contact a doctor if you are concerned about anything. You should also contact a doctor before you embark on a detox if you are on pharmaceutical medication.

You should not fast if you are pregnant, breastfeeding, diabetic, have liver or kidney disease, or if you are anaemic. It is not safe for small children to fast either.

DURING THE DETOX

It is fine to make the juices in the morning, or even the day before, ready to take in to work. Make sure you store them in the fridge and they will be fine for 24 hours. I prefer to store my juices in glass bottles. If you can't, then use BPA-free bottles instead (BPA is a compound found in plastics that is now believed to contribute to all sorts of health problems, so it's best to avoid it, if you can).

If making 4 different juices a day is too much for you, you can make 2 of the juices in the plans and double the recipes instead. The morning juices are supportive to the liver and detoxification, while the afternoon juices are more focused on nourishment and making sure there is a rich supply of nutrients for the body during the process. So choose one of each for the best detox experience.

It is a good idea to get organized with all the ingredients before you start. Doing this also gives you a bit of mental preparation for the process you are about to embark on. If you are making all the juices for the day in the morning, you can simply pour water through the juicer while it is still running until the water runs clear and then start on the next juice. It is not necessary to completely clean the juicer in-between each juice—make it as easy as you can!

While you are fasting, it is beneficial to dry body brush. It helps to remove the dead skin and the toxins. You may also find you get a coating on your tongue, so either get a tongue scraper or give your mouth a good rinse regularly through the day.

I have given smoothie options at certain points of the day because I do understand that it can be quite hard sometimes and you may need something a little bit more substantial to keep you sane! Doing a "liquid day" is a good alternative to a just juice day and is easier to cope with. The action of chewing sets your digestion process off, and by not doing that on just juice days we give the digestive system a rest. So yes, if you are having a smoothie, the gut will need to work a bit, but you are still getting massive benefits.

1-DAY DETOX—MAINTENANCE

The aim of doing a detox for a full day is to give the digestive system a rest and to reduce toxins in the body. It can be done weekly as a way of helping your liver deal with the onslaught of toxins that surreptitiously invade us in everyday life, whether from atmospheric pollution or the toxins we bring into our system, such as coffee, sugar, alcohol, tobacco, and many medications.

It is essential to be aware that it is not safe to fast while taking certain medications, and you should consult your doctor if you are unsure.

I would recommend weekly fasting if you are suffering from sluggishness and want to feel generally brighter.

What you need

2 apples
2 pears
1 small papaya
raspberries
2 lemons
2 limes

2 carrots
3 stalks of celery
lacinato kale
spinach
kale
cabbage

parsley
1 piece of fresh ginger
    ground turmeric

for the 3pm juice
raspberries
blueberries
strawberries
1 carrot
1 fennel bulb
parsley

OR for the 3pm smoothie
oats
blueberries
1 avocado
2 cups coconut water
chlorella powder
    or spirulina

The way we do it:

The recipe	When	Why
No.3 Turmeric Dream (page 20)	Between 6:30 am and 9:30 am	This is a great morning juice to wake the liver up and tell it that today we are going to help it deal with all the baddies in our body!
No.7 Super Green (page 26)	Between 11:30 am and 1:30 pm	You should still be feeling fine . . . so we are going to have a green juice for its detoxifying nutrients, encouraging the body to keep ridding itself of toxins.
No.83 Berry Boost (page 146) OR No.51 I Heart You (smoothie) (page 91)	Between 3 pm and 4 pm	Your energy may be dipping, and suddenly a single day feels like an eternity. If you have got this far, you are doing great! Our third juice contains more fruit for a bit of an energy boost. I have given a smoothie option here too. If you are really struggling, a smoothie is more substantial. You are still sticking to liquids without losing your mind and, let's face it, life is too short to be miserable. A liquid day is absolutely fine—you can work up to using just juices.
No.12 A Bit of Papaya (page 33)	Between 6 pm and 8 pm	You are nearly there. Have this gut-healing juice, relax, and sleep. You will have given your body a real helping hand, and it will thank you for it.

2-DAY DETOX—MONTHLY

This detox can be done each month. It goes slightly deeper and is useful if you prefer something more intense or find doing a day each week too difficult.

Because it takes slightly longer, I suggest reducing coffee, dairy, sugar, and alcohol in the preceding week. Eating a clean diet before the detox gives the system a head start because toxins will have already started being released. It also reduces the risk of headaches and side effects.

What you need

2 apples
1 pear
½ pineapple
1 orange
strawberries
blueberries
4 lemons

6 carrots
7 stalks of celery
1 cucumber
dandelion leaves
    (or spinach)
1 head of broccoli
1 globe artichoke
3 beets and their leaves
spinach
red or white cabbage

ground turmeric
acai berry powder
1 piece of fresh ginger
blue green algae

for the Day 1
3pm juice
1 nectarine
1 orange
1 carrot
1 sweet potato
ground cinnamon
flaxseed oil

OR for the Day 1
3pm smoothie
1 banana
1 pear
½ cup unsweetened almond
    milk (or filtered water)
maca powder
chamomile tea
pumpkin seeds

for the optional Day 2
mid-morning juice
2 oranges
1 lemon
wheatgrass juice or
    wheatgrass powder

for the Day 2
3pm juice
2 apricots
raspberries
2 carrots
spring greens
ground turmeric

OR for the Day 2
3pm smoothie
1 banana
blueberries
strawberries
sunflower seeds
flaxseeds
chlorella powder or spirulina
maca powder
1½ cups unsweetened
    almond milk (or filtered
    water)

The way we do it:

DAY 1		
The recipe	**When**	**Why**
No.3 Turmeric Dream (page 20)	Between 6:30 am and 9:30 am	Waking up the system to get the juices flowing to begin detoxification.
No.91 Feeling Light (page 158)	Between 11:30 am and 1:30 pm	This delicious juice will uplift, hydrate, elevate your mood, and keep you positive!
No.30 Happily Focused (page 61) OR No.21 Chill (smoothie) (page 50)	Between 3 pm and 4 pm	Because people often struggle around mid-afternoon, I suggest a smoothie option to help bridge the gap. It can be taken at this time on each detox day. You might have to work up to juice-only days, but even if you don't, liquid days are just as good. This juice and smoothie will both give you a bit of a boost.
No.50 Feeling Candy (page 90)	Between 6 pm and 8 pm	Congratulations! You've reached the end of day 1—it's quite an achievement! Have a final juice, and I wish you sweet dreams!

By day 2, you should wake up feeling pretty good, and surprisingly less hungry than you may have imagined.

DAY 2		
The recipe	**When**	**Why**
No.8 Liver Cleanse (page 27)	Between 6:30 am and 9:30 am	We start day 2 with a green juice that supports the liver as it detoxes.
OPTIONAL EXTRA No.32 Sweet Dream Shot (page 65)	Between juices 1 and 2	This is a great additional aid for sleep, but also a fabulous aid for cleansing. If you are feeling fine and so inclined, it is a nice addition to the second-day detox.
No.99 Rainbow Juice (page 168)	Between 11:30 am and 1:30 pm	A slight vitamin boost to make sure you have all the nutrients that your body needs during this process.
No.84 Sparkle and Shine (page 147) OR No.98 Nutrient Power (smoothie) (page 167)	Between 3 pm and 4 pm	You are almost there! If you feel fine, that's great, but if you are struggling, be sure to use the smoothie suggestion.
No.11 Tummy Help (page 32)	Between 6 pm and 8 pm	This final juice is a gentle soother for the gut. At the culmination of 2 days of fasting, your intestines will thank you for a bit of love.

3-DAY DETOX—EVERY 6 MONTHS

Focus and commitment are needed to do a juice fast for 3 days. If you have concerns about your health, I would advise that you check with your doctor before embarking on it. It is quite intense doing 3 days, but the benefits are huge, and you will feel like a different person by the end of it. You need to plan ahead and set aside a good time to do it. I recommend doing a 3-day fast once every 6 months.

If you can continue to work and go about a busy schedule as normal, then you can start your fast midweek. However, I advise starting on a Friday morning and ending on Monday morning, because allowing yourself time to sleep and relax is an essential part of the process. I would recommend a yoga session and maybe a massage for you to look forward to on days 2 and 3.

You will be going even deeper with this detox, and it is really important that you give yourself a head start and eat a clean diet full of nutrient-dense ingredients beforehand, which means no dairy, refined sugar, caffeine, or alcohol for at least a week before. Eat a diet full of vegetables and fruits, lean proteins, healthy fats, and complex carbs. The body needs to be stocked with nutrients that will support you and your liver during the coming detox.

What you need

1 pineapple
2 apricots
3 plums
1 watermelon
4 pears
1 papaya
1 banana
6 apples
blackberries
strawberries
blueberries
frozen blueberries
    or raspberries
raspberries
3 lemons
5 limes

lacinato kale
spinach
kale

10 stalks of celery
1 beetroot
2 carrots
Swiss chard
2 cucumbers
1 fennel bulb
dandelion leaves

mint
parsley
cilantro
4 pieces of fresh ginger
fresh/ground turmeric
ground cinnamon

wheatgrass juice or
    wheatgrass powder
mixed green powder
blue green algae
maca powder

chlorella powder
spirulina
flaxseed or evening primrose
    oil
sunflower seeds
ground flaxseeds
pumpkin seeds
sprouted sunflower seeds
aloe vera juice
½ cup unsweetened almond
    milk

**for the optional Day 2 & 3
mid-morning juice**

4 oranges
2 lemons
wheatgrass juice or
    wheatgrass powder

The way we do it:

DAY 1		
The recipe	**When**	**Why**
No.40 Wheatgrass Power (page 78)	Between 6:30 am and 9:30 am	We are going to start our 3-day journey by employing a juice to wake up and dazzle our system.
No.7 Super Green (page 26)	Between 11:30 am and 1:30 pm	This is a liver-oriented juice. We need to give really effective support to the liver when we are detoxing. This juice does just that.
No.16 Get Moving (smoothie) (page 37)	Between 3 pm and 4 pm	Because we are doing 3 days, I am putting in a fiber-rich smoothie at this time of the day. Not just because I know that it is hard to do 3 days on juice alone, but more importantly because we want the waste in the bowel and colon eliminated as quickly as possible. This is where the fiber helps.
No.99 Rainbow Juice (page 168)	Between 6 pm and 8 pm	This is a good all-around juice, giving a well-balanced spectrum of phytonutrients.

So, day 2! Hopefully you slept really well. People tend to feel surprisingly better in the morning than they expected, and much more positive about the day ahead.

DAY 2		
The recipe	**When**	**Why**
No.57 Supergreen Immune Support (page 105)	Between 6:30 am and 9:30 am	Green juice is the order of the day, with all its sulfur-forming vegetables that help the detox pathways in the liver. This juice has added vitamin B to keep us calm and nourish our nervous system.
OPTIONAL EXTRA No.32 Sweet Dream Shot (page 65)	Between juices 1 and 2	You can have this between juice 1 and 2, if you would like. If you are feeling fine and are so inclined, it is a nice addition to the second and third day of this detox.
No.70 Time for Turmeric (page 122)	Between 11:30 am and 1:30 pm	This juice is excellent all around and has anti-inflammatory actions—great for the body while it releases toxins.
No.47 Beyond Balanced (smoothie) (page 87)	Between 3 pm and 4 pm	Again, I have given a smoothie at this time of day. This is aimed at balancing energy levels, while nourishing you.
No.14 Calm Yourself (page 35)	Between 6 pm and 8 pm	A gut-soothing drink at the end of day 2 to help calm your tummy.

You are two-thirds of the way through—it is just one more day. I hope you have booked something nice to do today. If you are feeling a bit fatigued or have a head-ache, don't worry, these are normal during a detox as the body gets rid of toxins.

DAY 3		
The recipe	**When**	**Why**
No.4 Lime Parsley Punch (page 21)	Between 6:30 am and 9:30 am	A green alkalizing juice to start your day today.
OPTIONAL EXTRA No.32 Sweet Dream Shot (page 65)	Between juices 1 and 2	You can have this between juices 1 and 2, if you would like. Again, if you feel like it, this shot of goodness is a lovely thing to include.
No.48 On an Even Kale (page 88)	Between 11:30 am and 1:30 pm	I have chosen this juice to keep you going through the last day. It will give you a boost, and you should be feeling very proud of yourself, as well as starting to feel reenergized and lighter mentally and physically.
No.87 Skin Healer (smoothie) (page 152)	Between 3 pm and 4 pm	Today's smoothie is full of antioxidants and healing phytochemicals to make you glow.
No.13 Bloat Away! (page 34)	Between 6 pm and 8 pm	This is your final juice! I am sure the detox has had its ups and downs, but when you wake up tomorrow I am pretty sure that you will feel a whole lot better than you did before you started! To finish with is this lovely juice—again great for the gut.

GLOSSARY

Welcome to the Glossary—I hope you find this helpful. I have explained the benefits of each ingredient and in some cases suggested alternatives to use if you are having trouble finding certain things. You don't want to waste any produce or find an ingredient just doesn't agree with your taste buds and not have an alternative! Experiment—you will find a description of how the different fruit and vegetables can help your body. Have a look and you can create your own super juice or smoothie that suits your unique needs, helping you to get to know your body and your produce!

Acai Berry Powder Acai berries grow in large bunches at the top of acai palms in the Amazon rain forest. Packed with antioxidants, amino acids, fiber, essential fatty acids, vitamins, and minerals, acai berry powder is great for energy levels and for boosting your immunity. Because it has such high antioxidant levels, it is also fantastic for the reduction of free radicals. It comes in powder form, which is what I prefer to use, but you can get capsules and a liquid too.

Alfalfa Sprouts Because they are just sprouted, they contain a concentrated amount of vitamins, minerals, and enzymes, including calcium, potassium, magnesium, and vitamins C and K. They are great for energy levels and also can help with cholesterol levels. They are very nutrient-dense and are good to add to anything. You can buy or sprout your own alfalfa seeds on a damp piece of tissue much like cress—either is fine. If you don't have, or can't find, alfalfa then you can use other sprouted seeds, such as sunflower.

Almonds A source of good fats and antioxidants, good for your cholesterol and to help prevent cardiovascular disease. They contain vitamins E and K and magnesium, making almonds good for sleep and stress problems, calcium, and iron.

Almond Milk It's so easy to make at home. Put 1 cup (125 g) whole almonds and 3 cups (750 ml) water into a blender and whiz up then strain the liquid to remove the almond pulp. Almond milk has the same benefits as almonds. It is a great alternative to dairy as it has a similar consistency to milk and adds creaminess to smoothies.

Aloe Vera Great for many things, it is very soothing internally and fab for digestion, acid reflux, and IBS, as well as the immune system. A good source of vitamins A, C, E, B1, B2, B3, and B6, it even has a bit of B12! It also contains calcium, magnesium, zinc, chromium, selenium, sodium, iron, and potassium, as well as being packed with amino and fatty acids. Aloe vera comes in a liquid, so it is easy to add to your drinks.

Apple The juice has lots of fructose (fruit sugar), which gives the body instant energy. Its water content is high to help hydrate the body, and it's packed with flavonoids, all of which help mop up free radicals. Apples can be very helpful to people suffering with hay fever and asthma because they contain the phytonutrient quercetin. They also have a good amount of pectin, a type of soluble fiber, which is important for the transit of waste out of the body. Also high in vitamin C.

Apricot A good source of soluble fiber, they are also a good source of iron, potassium, and betacarotenes such as lycopene and lutein. Lycopene is good for hardening of the arteries, while lutein is great for the eyes and helpful for preventing macular degeneration. Both of these betacarotenes can be found in a lot of orange fruit and vegetables, such as apricots, sweet potatoes, and oranges.

Artichoke These contain inulin, which is great for blood sugar balance, and is also supportive to the liver because it contains compounds that are very protective. High in vitamins A, Bs, and C and potassium, manganese, biotin, and chromium. Artichokes also contain iodine, making them a helpful ingredient to include if you suffer from hypothyroidism.

Arugula It has glucosinolates, which are strong antioxidants that are supportive for detoxification and the liver. It is a bitter-tasting leaf, which helps the digestive juices flow, and it contains vitamins A, C, and folic acid and manganese, calcium, magnesium, copper, iron, and zinc.

Asparagus Boosts levels of enzymes that break down alcohol, and can act as a diuretic. Asparagus also has phytochemicals that have an anti-inflammatory effect. It contains vitamins A, C, K, and Bs, and potassium, sodium, and iron. It also has a high amount of protein for a vegetable.

Avocado When it comes to nutrition, avocados are in a class by themselves because of the unusually large number of benefits they offer. They are loaded with fiber and high in vitamins K, B1, B2, B5, B6, B9,

C, and E, betacarotene, potassium, lutein, and good fats, making them great for skin and hair health. They are a slow-burning fuel, so are useful for workout and post-workout energy levels. They are also amazing all around and a welcome addition to smoothies.

Banana   Bananas are great for lots of things, including insomnia, stress, blood pressure, and mood boosting, and the fiber can help with constipation and also help remove toxins during a healthy weight loss plan. They are high in fiber, potassium, tryptophan, manganese, and some copper, vitamin B6, vitamin C, betacarotenes, and lutein. They do have high fructose levels—the riper they are, the higher the natural sugars are.

Beet   Full of phytonutrients that have a high antioxidant and anti-inflammatory power. They help the liver with phase 2 detoxification, which is where toxins are bound to particles ready for excretion from the body. They also have high levels of iron, vitamins A, C, and B9, and magnesium, potassium, and betacyanins.

Blackberries   High in antioxidants, vitamin C, and also flavonoids, these berries are great for your skin and your gut. If there aren't any fresh ones around, see if you can get frozen ones, or substitute with raspberries or blueberries.

Blueberries   These are packed with antioxidants, anthocyanidins, and also vitamins B2 and C, soluble fiber and manganese. They are useful for eye- and age-related macular degeneration.

Blue green algae   Plant-like organisms found in both saltwater and freshwater lakes. This algae is high in protein, B vitamins, and iron and is great for boosting metabolism as well as immune system, bowel, and gut health.

Broccoli   A member of the cabbage family, broccoli contains glucosinolates, which help the excretion of estrogen from the body and are also antibacterial. The lutein in broccoli may be helpful in age-related macular degeneration. Broccoli is also high in vitamins C and A, folic acid, potassium, and fiber. The only time that raw broccoli shouldn't be used is when you suffer with an underactive thyroid, or hypothyroidism, though if you steam the broccoli first then you could juice or blend this.

Cabbage   "King" of the cruciferous family. Cabbage contains the notable phytochemical that is thought to have anti-cancer properties: indole-3-carbinol. The glucosinolates increase antioxidant protection and help to detoxify harmful chemicals and hormones. Cabbage juice is great for peptic ulcers and "leaky gut" because of the glutamine in it.

Cardamom   Similar to ginger and cinnamon, it is good for digestion and is stimulating for your circulation.

Carrot   High in betacarotene, a powerful antioxidant, which as a type of vitamin A helps eye health, reproduction, skin, and growth and development. Carrots are also rich in minerals and B vitamins, which help the metabolism.

Cayenne Pepper   It is anti-inflammatory, thermogenic, and good topically for skin conditions and effective for headaches. Also great for IBS, ulcers, and heartburn.

Celery   Hydrating and can act as an electrolyte. It also has coumarins, which may help to lower blood pressure. Really good for cholesterol. It is high in magnesium, potassium, calcium, and vitamins A and Bs.

Chard   High in lots of phytonutrients, especially carotenes and soluble fiber. It is good for bone health, and great for the colon. Also high in vitamins C, E, B, and K, fiber, chlorophyll and magnesium, potassium, iron, manganese, calcium, and selenium. Chard is dark green and these sorts of leaves are high in B6, so are great for PMS tenderness and balancing menstrual hormones. If you can't find chard, spinach is a good alternative.

Cherries   A great source of lots of flavonoids, especially anthocyanadins. These help inflammation, and are great for the treatment of gout. Cherries contain melatonin, so can be an effective sleep inducer. High in vitamins A, C (sweet cherries contain more), and E, melatonin, flavonoids, manganese, and copper.

Chia Seeds   These black seeds are a great source of fiber, protein, omega 3 and 6, vitamins B1, B2, and B3, and a really good amount of magnesium and manganese as well as zinc, potassium, and phosphorus. By soaking the seeds they absorb ten times their weight in water, making them fantastically hydrating when you add soaked chia to a smoothie or a juice (see page 187 for notes on soaking). The minerals in chia are great for bones and teeth, and chia is also good for insulin resistance, and making the body more sensitive to it. The fiber helps to remove toxins from the body, so it's good when detoxifying.

Chile Pepper   Gives you fire in your belly and by doing so helps lots of different ailments, including inflammation, congestion, and general low immunity. It is also thermogenic, making it a good metabolism boost if you are trying to lose weight.

Chlorella   A single-cell algae that is fantastic for the detoxification of toxins, including mercury. It is boosting to the body, especially the immune system, blood sugar balancing, and balancing the body's pH. It also helps to detoxify heavy metals. Chlorella comes as a green powder, which makes it easy to add to drinks. You can use it with other green powders such as spirulina and wheatgrass powder or on its own. Other green powders can also be substituted for chlorella.

Cilantro   Often used for detoxing heavy metals from the body. The cilantro binds to the heavy metals and mercury, in particular, in the body, and then the heavy metals are excreted. Cilantro is also high in selenium, chlorophyll, and B vitamins.

Cinnamon   Helps to regulate blood sugar, making it helpful for diabetics and people who suffer from insulin resistance. It can also help with yeast infections, stomach bugs, IBS, inflammation and antioxidants, and is good for triglyceride levels.

Coconut Water   Very hydrating, especially after exercise, and a great liquid to use in smoothies. It has a high potassium content, so is a good electrolyte drink.

Cucumber   Very hydrating, so good for skin, but also hydrating for all cells in the body. It has a good amount of vitamin K and antioxidants and is high in potassium and low in sodium. Cucumbers contain silica, which is good for joint pain.

Dandelion   It is high in nutrients and is great for liver function, weight loss, and blood sugar control. It is also a strong diuretic, which is helpful for any water retention. It is considered a digestive tonic because it is bitter and so helps the production of bile. And as a prebiotic, it is helpful for the good bacteria in your gut. It can be hard to find dandelion leaves or roots—try health food stores. However in the spring they can be found everywhere, so pick them from your garden! You can eat all parts, but for our purposes the leaves and the root are the most beneficial. If you cannot find any dandelions, use arugula or watercress instead.

Fennel   Amazing for the intestine, prebiotic, anti-spasmodic, and calming, while the phytoestrogens are good for the menopause and periods. Fennel is a good anti-inflammatory as it is good at interrupting inflammatory signaling. It is a good source of vitamin C and folic acid, as well as having decent amounts of magnesium, manganese, iron, calcium, and phosphorus.

Fig   High in soluble fiber, potassium, magnesium, calcium, iron, copper, and manganese. Figs are great for the intestines and also blood pressure. They are also very alkalizing.

Flaxseeds and Flaxseed Oil (also known as Linseed)   Flax helps with hormone balancing and inflammation. It is a good source of vegan omega 3s and is also high in fiber and lignans (phytoestrogens), potassium, magnesium, manganese, iron, and copper. They are small golden brown seeds. When they are pressed you get the oil, and this can be added to a juice or smoothie or used in salad dressings.

Garlic   It is known as nature's penicillin or nature's antibiotic and is a good immune booster. Great for blood pressure and cholesterol, it helps to reduce the potentially damaging LDL cholesterol while the protective HDL cholesterol levels remain unchanged. It is high in enzymes and sulfur-containing compounds. It is antimicrobial and protective against colon cancer and also helps with gut complaints. High in vitamins B6, C, and K and potassium, calcium, iron, and copper.

Ginger   Reduces nausea and eases indigestion, it is fantastic for the gut. Ginger is good for inflammation and can act as a painkiller. It is an immune-system boost and is a prebiotic, meaning it helps good colonies in the gut develop and aids a healthy transit through the digestive tract.

Grapes   Apart from the fact they make wine, the antioxidants and flavonoids in grapes are good for blood vessels and vascular conditions such as varicose veins. They contain vitamins A, B1, B2, C, and E and are a good source of potassium, phosphorus, and manganese.

Green Beans   Thought to be helpful for macular degeneration and a good antioxidant that is also supportive for cardiovascular health. They contain carotenoids including quercetin, kaempferol, catechins, vitamin C, betacarotenes, and manganese. They have a small but good amount of omega 3 alpha linolenic acid.

Hemp Seeds and Hemp Seed Oil   Good for energy levels and metabolic rate, hemp seeds can help lower cholesterol, manage blood pressure, and improve circulation and organ function. Can also help PMS. Hemp is good for hair and skin, having an anti-aging effect, and it can reduce inflammation and help immunity levels. It contains some protein, is a good vegan source of omega 3 and 6, and gamma-linolenic acid and is high in vitamin E. You can add hemp seeds to smoothies and sprinkle on top of food and the oil is good for smoothies and juices too. You could use flaxseed oil if you don't have hemp.

Himalayan Crystal Salt   This salt is from an evaporated primeval sea, and because it has been in the rocks for millions of years, it has a much higher mineral content than normal table salt. The human body needs to have salt to maintain healthy cell function and nerve conduction. It can also act as an electrolyte.

Honeydew Melon   It has a high water content and is good for skin, collagen, and tissue repair because it is high in vitamins C and B and copper.

Kale (Lacinato or Other Type)   A nutrient powerhouse, it is great for bones as it has a high calcium-to-phosphorus ratio. It is also an excellent source of chlorophyll and carotenes, betacarotene and lutein, and contains vitamins C, B1, B2, B6, and E, manganese, copper, iron, and calcium. If you don't like kale try kohlrabi leaves instead.

Kiwifruit   Have a good amount of antioxidants and enzymes and are helpful for respiratory problems, night coughing, and wheezing. They contain vitamins C, A, and E, and magnesium, potassium, copper, and phosphorus.

Lemon   Helps soothe your stomach and adds vitamin C to the mix. It also contains limonene, which is an important phytochemical, as well as folic acid and potassium. Lemons are alkalizing to the body even though they taste acidic.

Lime   Contains vitamin C and flavonoids called limonoids, such as limonene glucoside, which have antioxidant, anticarcinogenic, antibiotic, and detoxifying properties.

Maca Powder   A superpowder that has been used in Peru to help endurance, hormone levels, and energy levels, it is a great mood booster too. Contains potassium, iron, manganese, calcium, zinc, and copper.

Mango   Good for many things, including the cardiovascular system and infection. Mangoes are high in fiber, soluble and insoluble, as well as antioxidants, carotenoids, and a variety of phytochemicals. Mangoes contain vitamins A, C, B1, B6, folic acid, and E, and copper and magnesium.

Matcha Green Tea Powder   This powder is made from green tea leaves that are dried and ground into powder, making it very concentrated and packed with antioxidants that help the body in many ways: it can boost metabolism, help detoxification, is immune boosting, helps energy levels, boosts your mood, and helps with concentration. Contains fiber, vitamin C, selenium, chromium, zinc, and magnesium.

Milk Thistle   Milk thistle is a flowering herb that is in the daisy family. It is native to Mediterranean countries. It is the most well-known liver-supporting herb. Silymarin is the active ingredient and can also be found in artichokes, beet greens, and cilantro. It comes in a tincture (liquid), so the measurements used in the book are in drops.

Mint   Great for digestive issues, mint helps with gas and spasms in the gut. It relaxes the smooth muscle, therefore making spasms less. Helps with IBS. A powerful antioxidant.

Nectarine   See Peach

Oats   These are good for lowering cholesterol levels as they contain beta glucan, which helps remove cholesterol from the body. Oats are soothing to the gut, high in fiber, and slowly release energy to keep blood-sugar levels balanced. They are rich in B vitamins, selenium, phosphorus, magnesium, and calcium.

Soak oats for at least 30 minutes or overnight before adding to your smoothie. Do the same with chia seeds too. It is easier to soak oats/seeds in batches: soak 1 cup (100 g) of oats or 1 cup (150 g) chia seeds in 3 cups (750 ml) of cold water. When you're ready to use, drain the soaked oats/seeds and discard the water.

Orange   Excellent for overall health, a good immune booster, great for the connective tissues, helpful for cholesterol problems, and also helps fight viral infections, oranges have a good amount of vitamin C, but also a lot of flavonoids, including hesperidin. They also contain B vitamins including folic acid, carotenes, soluble fiber, and potassium.

Papaya   Has the digestive enzyme papain, which helps the digestion of proteins. It is a good antioxidant and great at dealing with free radicals. Contains carotenes, vitamins C, E, A, and folate, potassium, and fiber.

Parsley   Rich in chlorophyll and carotenes, parsley is great for helping the gut. It also has vitamin C, folic acid, magnesium, calcium, potassium, and zinc. It is often thought of as a stimulant and is a great energy source.

Passion Fruit   Can be helpful for blood pressure and is supportive to the cardiovascular and nervous systems. It can also help to increase blood production because it is high in vitamin C and iron. Passion fruit can assist with constipation as it acts as a mild laxative. Contains vitamin C, soluble fiber, iron, and potassium.

Peach   Contains lutein and lycopene, which are thought to be helpful for age-related macular degeneration and also may be helpful for heart conditions. Also contains carotenes, vitamin K, flavonoids, natural sugars, and insoluble fiber. You could use apricots or nectarines instead if you were having trouble getting hold of peaches.

Pear   The soluble fiber in pears helps the removal of any unwanted cholesterol. Pears contain vitamins C, B2, and E as well as potassium.

Pineapple   Contains vitamins C, B1, and B6, copper, magnesium, and fiber, as well as bromelain, a sulfur compound containing digestive enzymes, which also acts as an anti-inflammatory to the whole body.

Plum   High in antioxidants and fiber, they are often used for their laxative effect. Plums contain vitamins C and K and copper and potassium.

Pomegranate   Great for heart health, joint pain, inflammation, and overall health. It contains the antioxidants ellagitannin and anthocyanadins, as well as vitamin C.

Psyllium Husks   These act like a loofah in the bowel. Very fibrous, the husks will help get things moving if you need some help!

Pumpkin Seeds   These are helpful for many things including good prostate health because they contain phytosterols, in particular beta phytosterol, as well as essential fatty acids and a high level of magnesium, so they are soothing when we are tense and stressed out, as well as zinc, which will boost our immune system. They also have good levels of iron, manganese, zinc, and copper. Sunflower seeds would be a good alternative to pumpkin seeds.

Radishes   Great for liver disorders as they are a member of the cruciferous family and therefore high in sulfur compounds. Good for the gallbladder too. They contain vitamins C, B9, and K, molybdenum, calcium, and copper.

Raspberries   Nutrient powerhouses that have lots of flavonoids, mainly anthocyanidins, which are amazing antioxidants. Contains vitamins C, B2, and other B vitamins and manganese.

Red Pepper   Great source of vitamins C, E carotenes, B6, folic acid, B2, B3, B5, and K and potassium, magnesium, and phosphorus. A great source of antioxidant power, which is good for removing free radicals created when we are physically or mentally under stress.

Romaine Lettuce   The darker the lettuce, the higher the nutrient content it has. Romaine is a great source of chlorophyll, and vitamins A, C, B1, and B2, and also has a good amount of chromium and manganese. Mostly water, romaine lettuce is very hydrating and useful in juicing because of that. By all means use different varieties of lettuces. I like romaine because it is the most nutrient-dense of all the lettuce types.

Rosemary   Helpful for concentration and memory. It is very stimulating and has a high antioxidant activity. Great for inflammatory conditions and also digestion. Rosemary is amazing for colds and coughs, so try to include it more if you start to feel the first stages of illness.

Sage   Very useful for hot flashes during menopause, it is also antimicrobial.

Sesame Seeds   Great for digestion, circulation, and the intestines. They have a high protein content and contain good amounts of tryptophan, calcium, essential fatty acids, copper, magnesium, and iron.

Spinach   Useful for blood building and alkalizing the body, it is also helpful to detoxification and for the nervous system. Contains vitamins C and B (1, 2, 3, 6, 9), carotenes, and iron, magnesium, potassium, copper, and manganese.

Spirulina   A blue green algae superpowder, great for detoxing and alkalizing the body. It is also fantastic if you have any inflammation in the body. Rich in vegetable protein and B12 as well as betacarotene and iron, potassium, magnesium, sodium, phosphorus, and calcium. While spirulina is very similar to chlorella in lots of ways, spirulina has a higher protein and essential fatty acid content, while chlorella is better for detoxification due to a higher chlorophyll content. Having said that, if you don't have the right one in your cupboard, use the other one instead.

Spring Greens   Can help with inflammation, and can be protective against heart disease and stroke. They are high in indoles and sulfur and also contain vitamins C and K.

Strawberries   Because of their unique flavonoid content, they are great for inflammation. They contain vitamin B6, folic acid, biotin, B1, C, and K and are a very good source of manganese and iodine.

Sunflower Seeds   Good for inflammation and the immune system. This source of vegan protein contains vitamins E and B, magnesium, manganese, selenium, phosphorus, copper, iron, and fiber.

Sweet Potato   A great antioxidant and very good for the body. Helpful for blood sugar levels, sweet potatoes contain carotenes, vitamins B7 (biotin), B6, B5, B2, and C, and also the minerals manganese and copper.

Tomato   The carotenes in tomatoes are good for the skin, hair, eyes, and more serious inflammatory conditions, and the lycopene is thought to be very protective to the body, which is especially good for men and male hormones. Tomatoes contain vitamins C, K, B6, B5, B3, and folic acid as well as dietary fiber.

Turmeric Root   A wonderful anti-inflammatory spice, helpful to digestion and to flatulence, very supportive to the liver and therefore to detoxing the body. I love using fresh if I can, but it can be tricky to find, and ground is often more practical and just as good.

Watercress   This has many of the same properties as kale and arugula. Because of its bitter taste though, it is a stimulant for the release of bile and therefore aids the liver in the breakdown of fats.

Watermelon It is full of water, so is very hydrating while also being a great diuretic. It is also supportive to hormone balances in men. High in important antioxidants such as lycopene, high in vitamin C, and low in calories. Watermelons also contain vitamins A, B1, B6, and biotin and magnesium and potassium.

Wheatgrass A master detoxifier and cleanser. Very alkalizing, high in chlorophyll and vitamins A, C, and E and so supportive of the immune system. Great for energy levels and can help the metabolism because of the assistance it gives to the liver. Having said that, it also contains inositol, which is thought to be calming and relaxing so will help you sleep when your body needs it. Wheatgrass is the young grass of the wheat plant and grows in Europe and America. You can grow your own by soaking wheat seeds in water and cutting off the shoots! The powder comes from the grass being dried and ground. It is very concentrated and I like the powder to add to my drinks. Fresh is great, but not always practical! A **wheatgrass shot** is a small glass of juiced wheatgrass. It has a strong taste so drink it quickly or add it to juices and smoothies.

Zucchini Hydrating and high in potassium, carotenes, and vitamin C—good for skin, immunity, and gut health.

INDEX

INDEX

ACKNOWLEDGMENTS

The first people I would like to thank are my family; my husband, Jake, and my girls Elfie, Bliss, and Blythe, they have been my willing (most of the time) testers and tasters throughout the juicing of this book. I would also like to thank the rest of my family, who have been really patient and listened to me rambling on about food and nutrition for years and not just while writing this book!

Thank you to all at Storm Artists who have been trying out the juices in the office and giving honest feedback . . . most seem converted now!

This book looks good because we had a great creative team, David Eldridge the book designer, Nassima Rothacker, who took the beautiful pictures, Frankie Unsworth who juiced and juiced and juiced, Cynthia Inions for the lovely grays and blues.

Ebury publishing and especially Laura Higginson need a medal for actually letting me publish a book, and also guiding me through the process. I would also like to thank Rue Down for her invaluable advice.

And last but by no means least I need to acknowledge my girlfriends who are always a source of inspiration and, because they are a strong-headed bunch, have always got an opinion, which has been instrumental in getting me this far!